Aspiration and Injection Therapy In Arthritis and Musculoskeletal Disorders

Otto Steinbrocker, M.D.
Consulting Physician (Rheumatology)
Hospital for Joint Diseases and
Lenox Hill Hospital, New York, New York

David H. Neustadt, M.D.
Associate Clinical Professor of Medicine and
Chief, Section on Rheumatic Diseases,
University of Louisville School of Medicine,
Louisville, Kentucky

Aspiration and Injection Therapy In Arthritis and Musculoskeletal Disorders

A Handbook on Technique and Management

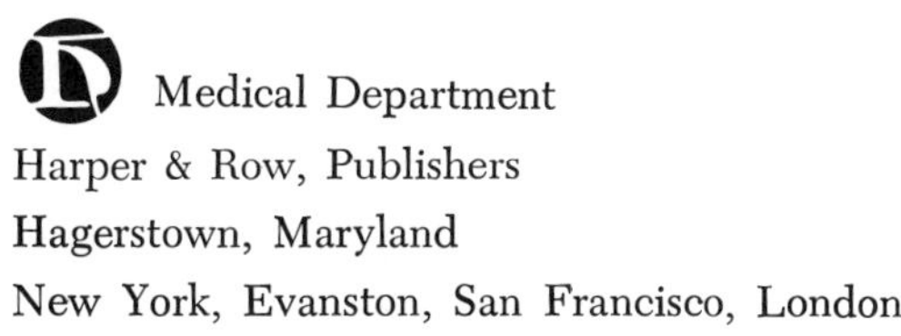

Medical Department
Harper & Row, Publishers
Hagerstown, Maryland
New York, Evanston, San Francisco, London

First edition

Standard Book Number: 06-142497-8

Library of Congress Catalog Card Number: 72-6318

Contents

Preface

The most common complaint in musculoskeletal disorders is pain—the symptom for which the patient most frequently seeks medical attention. It serves as the physician's chief guide in evaluating response. When pain continues unabated in the locomotor system, it often dominates the clinical picture and sometimes assumes the proportions of a disease in the patient's mind. Therefore, evaluation of pain and its effective relief take on great importance in many disorders. In arthritis and related conditions where pain is a chief symptom, acute or unresponsive to the usual measures, special methods of management become necessary.

Musculoskeletal pain associated with inflammation may be part of a complex of symptoms reflecting a systemic disorder. However, pain may arise from a localized lesion and resist the usual general or local measures. Sound diagnostic examination must be a primary consideration. Control of pain and/or suppression of inflammatory response may merely be an adjunct to a comprehensive management program. Fortunately, in many patients *local injections at the source of pain or tissue level frequently give prolonged relief or abolish the symptoms.*

In the course of many years teaching postgraduate courses in rheumatologic disorders and the problems of musculoskeletal pain, it has become obvious that two major considerations need emphasis: due recognition of the significant role of pain in the clinical picture and the application of an appropriate comprehensive treatment regimen.

This handbook is a readily available compilation of indications and techniques in which unnecessary discussion has been avoided. It should prove of great value to various clinicians desirous of increasing their resources and skills for the total care of painful musculoskeletal disorders—family physicians, internists, rheumatologists, physiatrists, neurologists, orthopedists, and pediatricians.

This volume describes local measures which we have found useful in daily clinical practice. With few exceptions, these procedures are widely used and generally accepted, but are sometimes practiced casually and often timidly because the techniques have not been taught or are only employed occasionally. Also some specific local and regional techniques of injection require special training.

The complete management of locomotor pain is greatly enhanced by the proper selection and administration of local or regional injections. The successful application of local injection and intrasynovial therapy requires an understanding of the diagnosis, accurate localization of pathology, and the choice of suitable injection techniques. Good judgment and skill come naturally with the enlightenment acquired by observation and application.

Aspiration and Injection Therapy In Arthritis and Musculoskeletal Disorders

1

Introduction

Treatment of musculosketal disorders by local or regional injection is indicated in acute disorders in which the condition is obvious and the patient needs relief (acute tenosynovitis or bursitis, synovitis with effusion) (Hollander, 1966), in refractory localized pain or as a supplement to a treatment program to speed overall improvement. Not infrequently injections of lidocaine or corticosteroid provide the additional aid which alone, or as an adjunct to the management program, overcomes the refractory pain (Hollander, 1966; Miller, 1956, 1957; Findler and Post; Neustadt, 1963; Steinbrocker, 1941). They are useful to initiate and facilitate physiatric regimens.

For the relief of local, circumscribed, musculoskeletal pain, analgesic injection therapy may be given by direct local infiltration of the tender site, as elicited by palpation with the fingertip (Hollander, 1966; Steinbrocker, 1941). It may be effective in many common lesions of soft tissues (Table 1). Only a few regional techniques have been found by the authors to be suitable for everyday practice without special training. Intrasynovial corticoid therapy has been found to be helpful (Hollander, 1970; Miller 1956, 1957; Neustadt, 1963).

ANALGESIC AGENTS

Analgesic preparations in aqueous solution are used.· (Table 2) The authors have found aqueous solutions of anesthetic compounds to be safe and frequently prolonged in their effects. We prefer to use lidocaine solution, 1 per cent or its equivalent (without epinephrine) (Steinbrocker, 1952; Hannington-Kiff). Procaine and other long-used local anesthetics

TABLE 1. Painful Nonarticular Rheumatic Disorders

Fibrositis
- Localized
  - Myalgia and myositis, fasciitis, tender point and "trigger" point syndromes, scapulocostal syndrome, Dupuytren's contracture
- Systemic
  - Myopathies, fibromyalgic syndrome (muscular rheumatism), polymyalgia rheumatica; myalgia, arthralgia, neuralgia, vasomotor instability

Bursitis
- prepatellar, olecranon, subdeltoid, etc.

Periarthritis
- adhesive capsulitis, scapulohumeral capsulitis, frozen shoulder

Tenosynovitis
- tendovaginitis ("snapping" finger), De Quervain's syndrome, bicipital, epicondylitis (tennis elbow)

Tendinitis
- calcareous bursitis (subacromial), of the hip, noncalcific tendinitis

Neuritis
- neuralgia, neuropathy

Reflex neurovascular dystrophy
- causalgia, Sudeck's atrophy, posttraumatic dystrophy, shoulder-hand syndrome

---

Any of the above may be primary, localized, specific or idiopathic; or associated with systemic disease.

are more likely to have been administered previously. A history of any untoward effect from a local anesthetic injection should be ascertained in advance. It is wise in any case to start with one of the newer compounds (Editorial, 1971). Patients sensitive to one compound may tolerate other anesthetic solutions, tested in small amounts (drops) in dilution, intracutaneously or preferably first on the skin. Many compounds are available and effective.

Corticosteroids in suspension in small quantity are added to facilitate and increase inadequate effects in extraarticular soft tissue disorders. Suspensions are preferred to provide gradual release of corticosteroid content with the anesthetic for immediate relief (Table 3).

Intraarticular injections were carried out with a variety of compounds for relief of symptoms long before the advent of corticosteroids. Un-

TABLE 2. Materials and Dosage (for Analgesic Injections)

Normal saline solution for control tests

Ethyl chloride spray (to freezing) for preliminary spot anesthesia or as local analgesia

Procaine, lidocaine (preferably) or equivalents, 1% *without* epinephrine, for preliminary skin wheal, as a control test or preceding deeper injection

- Dose
  - 1–20 ml 1% solution (without epinephrine)
  - No more than 5 ml of 0.5% at first injection
  - No more than 20 ml slowly, gradually increased (usually) for the ambulatory patient
  - Intervals of 3–7 days, occasionally daily for acute state

Corticosteroid

- Repository suspensions: hydrocortisone, prednisolone, triamcinolone, methylprednisolone and betamethasone (strength variable in each preparation)
- Dose dependent on lesion and site, contained in 0.125 to 3.0 ml

TABLE 3. Materials and Dosage (for Injection of Corticosteroids)

Lidocaine and corticosteroid mixtures*

Amounts according to site at intervals of 1 to 8 weeks or longer

Needles, 25 G, 0.5 in. for wheals; length for deep injections dependent on depth of lesion, 22 or 20 G

Repository Preparations (equivalent doses)	per ml	Range of usual dosage
Hydrocortisone Tebutate (TBA)	50 mg	25–100 mg
Prednisolone Tebutate (Hydeltra-TBA)	20 mg	5–40 mg
Betamethasone acetate and disodium phosphate (Celestone Soluspan)	6 mg	1.5–6 mg
Methylprednisolone acetate (Depo-Medrol††)	20 mg	4–80 mg
Triamcinolone acetonide (Kenalog, Aristocort)	20 mg	5–40 mg
Triamcinolone hexacetonide (Aristospan)	20 mg	5–40 mg

* The same precautions should be observed as with "caine" injections.

†† Supplied in: 20 mg per ml, 40 mg per ml, and 80 mg per ml preparations.

fortunately, none of the analgesic preparations available before cortisone had any durable effects. The introduction of intrasynovial corticosteroids has added a useful resource for the management of pain and inflammation in articular, bursal, tenosynovial disease, and other soft tissue disorders. It provides dependable and prolonged relief of joint symptoms producing increased functional capacity of the treated joints, as well as a suppressive effect on the inflammatory manifestations.

The judicious use of the newer corticosteroids and their suspensions make therapeutic injection of inflamed joints and various painful musculoskeletal conditions, a much more effective part of the management program. The duration of the results varies with the site and severity of involvement. Possible adverse reactions occur rarely from such treatment and must be weighed against the potential known benefits. The intervals between injections, the dosage used, and the total amount of the compound administered over a given time determine the relative soundness of the procedure. The longer the intervals the better; we usually recommend a 4 weeks' minimum for intraarticular procedures. The hazard of aseptic necrosis (osteonecrosis) must be considered, particularly when injections are given repeatedly at the hip and shoulder. In chronic disorders the prospects must be good for at least appreciable improvement of pain or function. Local injections into painful tissues should be carried out according to established principles of local analgesia (Table 4).

TABLE 4. Principles of Local Analgesia

1. Determination of point(s) of maximum tenderness (PMT) or trigger point
    a. palpation of symmetrical uninvolved area (for comparison) and affected part for localization
    b. palpation and needling of trigger points for reproduction of pain
    c. after injection of PMT with procaine solution, the pain, tenderness greatly improved or abolished within 5–15 minutes.
2. Areas of lesser tenderness not injected
3. Test for cutaneous hyperesthesia by scratch and pinch, over PMT and elsewhere, before injection
4. Skin wheal before deep injection
5. Control injection (subcutaneous) of normal saline soultion
6. Search for other PMT and reevaluate if relief inadequate after 2–3 injections of lidocaine

DOSAGE

Procaine-like Analgesics

Aqueous lidocaine solution is used in 1 per cent strength ordinarily, except for the 0.5 per cent administration used initially to test the patient's tolerance (see Table 2, page 3). The concentration may be increased thereafter. Procaine (Novocaine) and other anesthetic solutions are widely used and are as effective. Because of their almost univeral application, the likelihood of hypersensitivity is diminished by using a later formulation such as lidocaine, which also has a longer duration of action time (Steinbrocker, 1952; Hannington-Kiff). (In further discussion reference to "lidocaine solution," "anesthetic solution," or "analgesic solution" will mean 1 per cent solution of lidocaine [serocaine, Xylocaine] or equivalent.) Fresh, undeteriorated solutions are used at room temperature. We do not add epinephrine to any of the local analgesic or anesthetic solutions employed for relief of pain (see Table 2, page 3). The amount used at any session varies from 1 to 20 ml, depending upon the site of injection, the tolerance of the patient, and whether he is ambulatory.

It is customary to start with a small dose, to test the patient's tolerance, and then to increase the amount at each further treatment. In ambulatory patients it is unwise to administer more than 20 ml at any session without well-demonstrated tolerance. The large doses used in surgical anesthesia are not required. Those individuals who must drive cars or perform hazardous work after an injection need especially careful consideration in the use of these preparations and in the administration of barbiturates or other premedication. It is recommended that someone accompany the patient for the first one or two injections.

Corticosteroids

Corticosteroid dosage must be arbitrarily selected. Factors deserving consideration include the size of the joint, the severity of inflammation, previous response, the amount of strain from weight-bearing or other activity, and the systemic state.

For estimating dosage, a useful guide is as follows: for small joints of the hand and feet, 2.5 to 15 mg of prednisolone suspension or equivalent; for medium size joints such as the wrists and elbows, 10 to 20 mg; for the knee, ankle and shoulder, 20 to 50 mg; and for the hip 25 to 50 mg. Occasionally, it is necessary to give larger amounts to obtain optimum results.

Numerous hydrocortisone derivatives are available for intrasynovial administration (see Table 3). All of these agents can produce significant anti-inflammatory effect when given in adequate dosage directly into an inflamed joint. The major criterion to designate a preparation of first choice is longest duration of therapeutic effectiveness. Although some patients obtain greater beneficial effects from one steroid compound than another, no single steroid agent has shown a convincing margin of superiority over the others in controlled trials. (Neustadt 1963). If recent observations are confirmed, it would appear that the less soluble suspensions, triamcinolone hexacetonide (Aristospan) and betamethasone acetate (Celestone Soluspan) do prolong the beneficial therapeutic effect.

Number of Injections

If pain returns after an analgesic (caine) injection, usually with diminished intensity, the site may be reinfiltrated. The procedure may have to be repeated at intervals of a few days to 3 weeks or more, depending on the severity of the complaints and the rate of response. In extremely troublesome or acute conditions, local injection daily may be required for several treatments, before longer intervals suffice.

We have injected some individuals with analgesics only once, others 10 to 12 times, before obtaining satisfactory results. One patient required 16 injections before lasting relief was obtained. If no improvement of symptoms or signs occurs after 2 or 3 local injections in increasing amounts, discontinuance of treatment at that site and reevaluation of the patient is in order. It is generally accepted that about 5 per cent of individuals are refractory to procaine, probably also to lidocaine and similar compounds. Other local anesthetics may prove effective in these unresponsive patients, since the formula differs in each of these compounds.

MATERIALS

NEEDLES AND SYRINGES

Disposable needles and syringes are convenient and sterile. For those who give many injections and prepare their own equipment, autoclaving is the safest method of sterilization. Luer lock syringes and needles are useful. When long needles are used, the security type with beaded needle is desirable. The length of the needle varies from 0.5 to 4.0 in. according to the depth of the procedure to be carried out. The usual sizes adequate for the various approaches are listed below:

Intracutaneous skin wheal: 0.5 in., 25 G
Local intramuscular injections or tender point infiltrations: 1.5 to 2 in., 22 G
Arthrocentesis of knee: 2.5 in., 20 G
Deep gluteal or epidural injection: 3 to 4 in., 20 to 22 G

The gauge ordinarily used for parenteral injection is 22 or 20 G, preferably the former, in order to minimize discomfort. For the skin wheal a short 25-G needle is best. In unusual situations, or when thick fluid must be removed, as in a ganglion or cyst when inspissated material is expected, a 16- to 18-G needle may be necessary, after a skin wheal with lidocaine has been made. It is probably wise to use no syringe larger than 10 ml for injection of fluid or for aspiration or suction. It is easier to use a 10-ml syringe a few times with its lesser suction for aspiration, and its lower pressure for injection, than a larger one. The regular 2-ml, 5-ml, and 10-ml syringes suffice for these procedures. The Luer Lock syringe, for those who autoclave their equipment, provides a safety device that prevents spattering, when the syringe and needle happen to be loose, and prevents a sudden slipping of the needle from the syringe.

TABLE 5. The Standard Injection-Aspiration Tray (Quantities in Parentheses)

Sterile Tray (13 × 9 × 1 inches)

- Syringes, preferably Luer lock
  - 10 ml (3)
  - 5 ml (3)
  - 2 ml (3)
- Needles
  - 0.5 in., 25 G (3)
  - 1.5 in., 22 G (3)
  - 2.0 in., 22 G (3)
  - 2.0 in., 18 G (2)
  - 2.5 in., 20 G (3)
  - 2.5 in., 20 G (3)
  - 2.5 in., 22 G (3) security type c̄ safety bead
  - 4.0 in., 20 G (3) security type c̄ safety bead
- Towels (3)
- Hemostat or forceps

Additional items, as needed

- Tincture of iodine, pHisohex or other antiseptic solution
- Alcohol sponges (10)
- Lidocaine 1%, or other anesthetic solution (1 bottle)
- Normal saline solution (1 bottle)
- Band-Aids, gauze pads (6), and cotton tip applicators
- Tubes for culture, and synovial fluid analysis (EDTA 5 mg or heparin 1 or 2 drops are satisfactory anticoagulants)

The tray is kept sterile; the top portion autoclaved or containing disposable items.

TABLE 6. Synovial Fluid Examinations

Physical Studies*
- Quantity (ml)
  - Volume
- Appearance
  - Color
  - Clarity
- Viscosity
  - Estimate of "stringing" a drop of fluid; Ostwald viscosimeter
- Clot formation
  - (spontaneous)
- "Mucin" clot test
  - Qualitative measure of hyaluronate–protein

Microscopic Exam*
- Cytology
  - Total CBC and differential count
- Microscopic (light, polarizing and phase):
  - Crystal identification and inclusion cells (ragocytes)

Bacteriologic exam**
- Smear, Culture

Immunologic studies**
- Rheumatoid factor
- Antinuclear factor
- LE cells
- Total Complement level

Chemical studies**
- Glucose
  - Synovial fluid/plasma "difference" (simultaneous determination)
- Total Protein content
- Lactic Dehydrogenase level

Other Tests***
- pH determination
- Specific gravity
- Fibrinogen content
- Immunoglobulin analysis
- Other enzyme determinations

---

* Essential procedure (routine)
** May be of clinical value
*** Rarely of clinical value

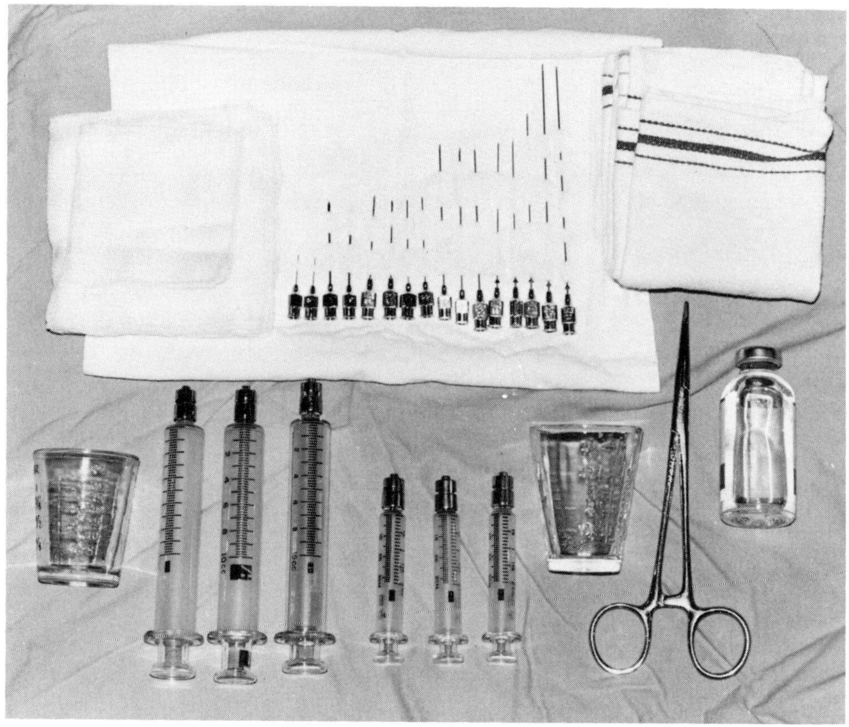

Fig. 1–1. The Aspiration-Injection Tray (see Table 5)

It is a great convenience to have a sterile aspiration-injection tray prepared and ready in the hospital, clinic or office (Fig. 1-1). It should contain the items needed for arthrocentesis and/or injection of any joint or site (Table 5).

Tests and procedures which are useful for analysis of aspirated synovial fluid are outlined in Table 6. Tests routinely performed are grouped with a single or double asterisk, and those considered special or generally less useful are marked with 3 asterisks. Table 7 lists the findings in normal fluid compared with those which may be found in pathologic fluid. In some cases, only a few drops of fluid may suffice to establish the diagnosis, especially for septic arthritis or a specific form of crystal synovitis (Cohen; Ropes & Bauer).

MECHANICAL INJECTORS

Mechanical trigger devices for cutaneous and deeper injection have recently become available. The authors have found that patients with hypersensitive skin, or those who find deeper needling unpleasant or

TABLE 7. Synovial Fluid Analysis

Technique or procedure	Interpretation	
	Normal	Pathologic Fluid
Gross appearance	Clear, pale yellow	Cloudy to opaque, yellow-green to gray
Viscosity	Viscous	Decreased viscosity or "watery"
Clot formation	Does not clot	Clots on standing
"Mucin" clot test	"Ropy," tight clot	Loose clot to shreds
Total WBC	<600	>2000
diff	Polys <25%	Polys>65%
Microscopic exam	No crystals	Crystals and inclusion cells
Bacteriologic exam	Sterile	
Immunologic studies rheumatoid factor antinuclear factor complement	Negative tests Normal complement level	May be positive tests Complement reduced
Glucose level	Same as blood	Blood/synovial fluid difference>30 mg%
Total protein content	Low	Increased
LDH activity	Normal level	Increased
pH determination	Alkaline	Usually acid

intolerable, are easily and more comfortably treated with these devices. They are useful aids in the hands of clinicians employing them often enough to acquire facility in their application. The instruments make injection therapy more versatile and better tolerated by sensitive and "needle shy" individuals. Unpleasant skin wheals produced by needle are annoying. Ethyl chloride spray anesthesia may be useful, but is not well tolerated by some patients.

The Dermo-Jet

This instrument consists of a relatively simple trigger-like arrangement whereby the medication in a storage compartment is forced into the skin in doses of 0.1 ml, and automatically released when the trigger is pressed (Fig. 1–2) (Steinbrocker, in preparation). The amount of pressure and the distance from the skin make an intracutaneous wheal when the liquid penetrates the outer layer of the cutis (Fig. 1–3). The authors use this device often for intracutaneous wheals of lidocaine. It provides so com-

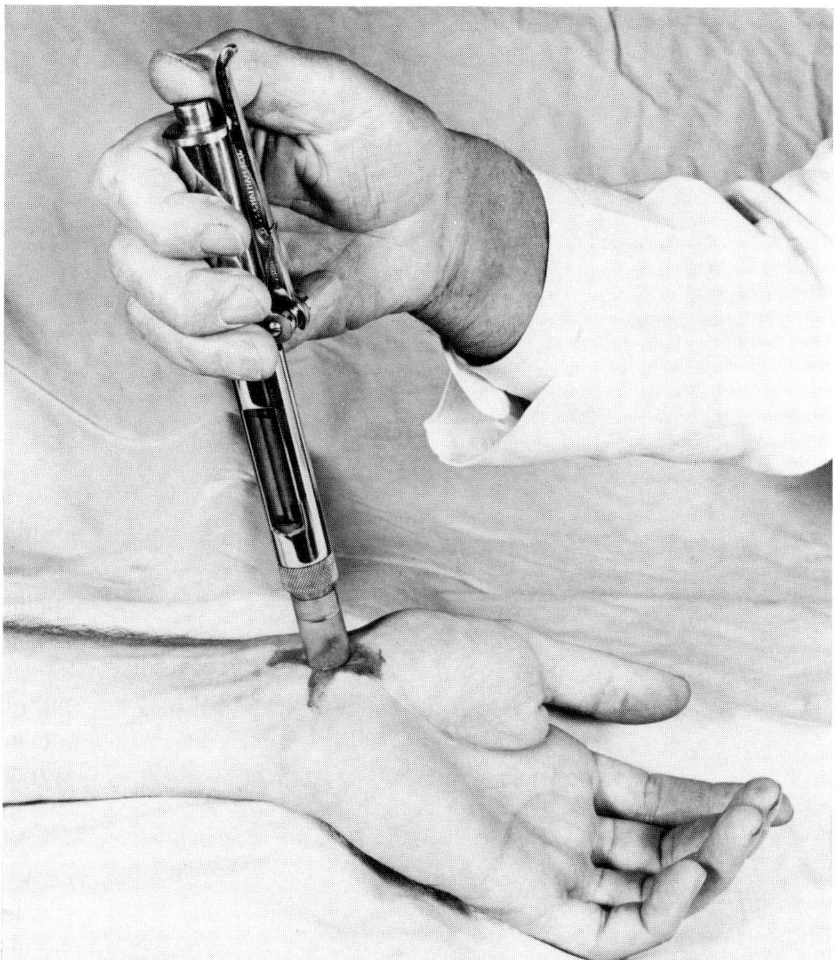

Fig. 1–2. The Dermo-Jet used as a wheal maker.

fortable an entry point for the patient that we rarely use a needle and syringe for skin wheals.

Deeper injection must be made through the wheal by the usual route for aspiration and intrasynovial or intramuscular injection. In overly sensitive or needle-shy individuals, the instrument makes withdrawal of venous blood a tolerable procedure by making a wheal over or preferably beside the vein for the site of needle entry.

Dermatologists have used this device for some time for intralesional injections of the skin, with corticoids and other drugs.

Application. The Dermo-Jet produces an anesthetic wheal nearly pain-

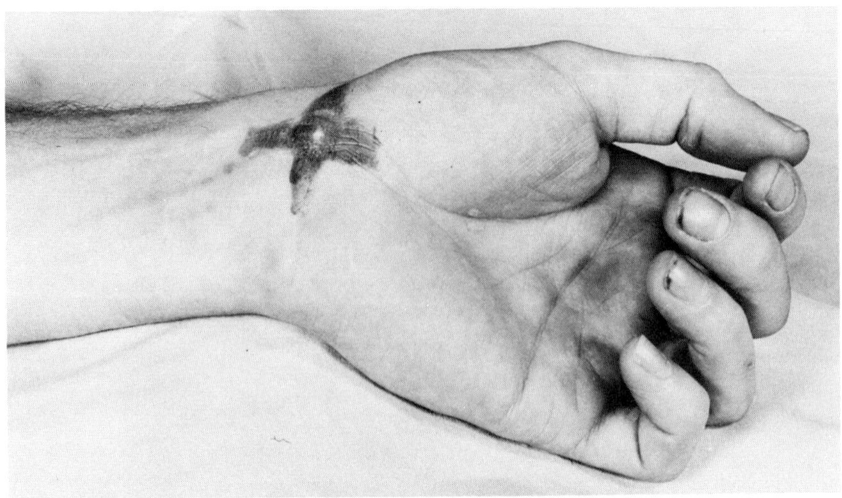

Fig. 1–3. Skin wheal produced by the Dermo-Jet.

lessly. For superficial tissues or joints the wheal is best made to one side of the inflamed or tender point such as a metacarpophalangeal joint, not at a bony prominence—that is, at the most padded area close to the point of entry. The needle then is advanced through the wheal into the swollen capsule or just over it and the injection is made. Some discomfort is produced by the latter maneuver, but the injection of small sites of inflamed tissue or joints is usually more comfortably carried out in this way than by conventional methods (hypodermic wheal or freezing the skin).

Limitations. There are no disturbing effects with the use of the Dermo-Jet. However, the patient should be told that there will be a relatively painless sound like that of a little firecracker or a stapler. In a few individuals with sensitive skin, ecchymosis has occurred. Occasionally, there is a slight oozing of blood where the pressure of the spray enters the skin.

Cleansing of a few parts and sterilizing are required every 48 hours; the rest of the instrument should be cleaned once a month.

There is no untoward effect from the repeated use of this device in the same area. Any material injected is deposited only within the skin for a wheal.

The Hypospray

The Hypospray is a more powerful and elaborate triggered instrument than the Dermo-Jet, with more versatile capacity for injections of ac-

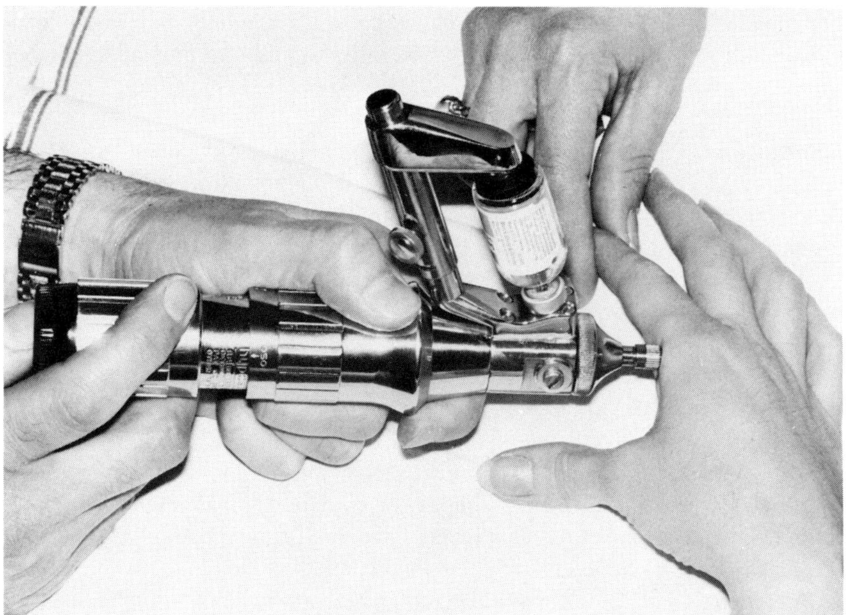

Fig. 1–4. The Hypospray placed for an intraarticular injection. Medication is ejected through the skin, underlying tissues, and into the joint in one step or spray.

cessible joints and musculoskeletal structures. It permits precise loading of a quantity of medication to be delivered up to 1 ml (Ziff *et al.*). Lidocaine, corticosteroid, or combinations may be given (Fig. 1–4). Any of these may be employed according to the patient's requirements, since the instrument permits a change of the medication as needed, preparations in standard rubber-capped vials are attached to the apparatus and readily interchanged.

When the trigger is pressed, the set measured amount of medication is forced through the cutis and underlying tissue for some distance. The pressure is sufficient to treat accessible articular, bursal, neural, and other lesions of soft tissues. The deeper joints, such as the hips, do not lend themselves to such treatment. Joints containing much fluid, such as effused knees, are usually not suitable for hypospray injection.

The Hypospray, by virtue of its dose-adjustable mechanism, and by attaching special tips, may be used for intracutaneous, intramuscular, or intraarticular injections into accessible joints. (It cannot be used for aspiration.)

It is a convenient, quick, and comfortable way of getting the medication in one step through the the skin into the tissues or joint to be injected.

For needle-shy subjects or children it proves especially useful by providing more comfortable administration of analgesic and antiinflammatory injections.

Limitations. The Hypospray requires daily care and cleansing for removal of drug residue. It requires meticulous attention to details, but these are quickly mastered. Someone must be assigned to the care of the instrument and the preparation of the medications, to insure sterile introduction of corticosteroids. At least monthly sterilization or autoclaving of certain parts is required.

Bleeding or oozing at the entry point when any preparation is forced through the skin is usually negligible. Application of pressure after the injection is helpful. Ecchymosis may rarely be extensive at the point of instrumental pressure.

Considerable transient discomfort may be experienced when the hypospray is applied at inflamed areas or over bony prominences. In such patients the approach to the joint or inflamed area must be made from the least sensitive adjacent point.

The instrument is not suitable for instramuscular or other musculoskeletal injections of tender areas requiring amounts of lidocaine greater than 1 to 3 ml (three injections).

When aspiration of a joint or bursa is necessary for examination of fluid the use of a needle and syringe becomes necessary.

2

Basis of Analgesic Injections

Although infiltrative, analgesic treatment is essentially palliative, it often provides striking and lasting relief of pain. Increased function of the part and general improvement may follow single or repeated injections. The benefits may last much longer than the duration of anesthesia. Such results raise the question of the basis of the prolonged effects. The clinical course of patients under treatment and their responses suggest a number of direct and indirect sources of amelioration. These are largely speculative, because the exact mechanism of lasting therapeutic analgesia has not been demonstrated or thoroughly clarified.

RATIONALE

The mechanism of response and relief probably is not identical in all cases; pain as well as disability may be quite diverse and variable. Most observers, however, give one or more of the following explanations: local hyperemia; relaxation of reflex muscular spasm (contraction); generalized systemic response following relief of local pain with increased rest and sleep, as well as a beneficial influence upon local tissue metabolism initiated by these local effects; modification of the pain threshold; and helpful mechanical effects from the introduction of the solution. The increased mobility permitted even for a short while as a result of the relief of pain undoubtedly accelerates recovery and function. Placebo therapy and "suggestion" often are mentioned. The high percentage of response and elimination of symptoms make these considerations inadequate, although it may be true in some cases, as has been shown by placebo testing.

Relief of muscular spasm or contraction is often mentioned and assumed in the pain of supportive tissues. This is a controversial subject. With suitable apparatus it is possible to confirm the concept and to demonstrate in some individual patients the presence of muscular contraction or of excessive neurostimulation. From a practical standpoint it is commonly observed that tender, firm muscles in a painful area or about a troublesome joint become relaxed and lose their soreness when a point of maximum tenderness is injected or when an area of deep tenderness is infiltrated. Some idea of the amount of muscular involvement, and the extent to which it is responsible for the symptoms, may be demonstrated by these procedures. The more that localized muscular irritability and contraction contribute to complaints, the greater the likelihood of effective relief by repeated analgesic injections. When significant organic changes are present, or when poor body mechanics are uncorrected, analgesic injections afford only transient relief and symptoms recur rapidly.

INDICATIONS

Diagnostic injections of analgesic solution may provide valuable aid in the scalenus anticus syndrome, subdeltoid bursitis, neuritides, and other complaints by confirming the localization and abolition of symptoms through regional intramuscular, peritendinous (bursal) or perineural injections. Paravertebral spinal nerve block or sympathetic ganglion block sometimes is required.

Therapeutic injection of analgesic substances is indicated when, after thorough examination, visceral disease has been ruled out as the source of pain, a "working" musculoskeletal diagnosis is made, there are local, accessible signs likely to respond to direct infiltration, and when the usual therapeutic methods have failed.

In traumatic, and in some inflammatory or degenerative processes of joints, periarticular and supporting tissues, especially in lesions of soft tissues at tender and trigger points (see Table 1, page 2) appropriate injection therapy frequently provides palliative and sometimes durable relief (Hollander, 1966; Miller, 1956; Findler & Post; Neustadt, 1963; Steinbrocker, 1952).

Acute, obvious conditions warrant immediate direct injection for rapid relief. Refractory, localized symptoms may respond to local or regional injection alone or as a supplementary measure.

CONTRAINDICATIONS

Hypersensitivity to any analgesic preparation disqualifies it and any derivative of the same formula.

Local injections should not be administered at infected sites or in the vicinity of infection.

Placebo infiltration of apprehensive or neurotic individuals, in whom a great part of the symptomatology may arise from emotional or psychologic factors, requires great care in the evaluation of the response.

HAZARDS

The most serious hazards in the use of local anesthetic or analgesic injections are hypersensitivity and accidental intravenous introduction. Serious, even fatal hypersensitivity to procaine and other anesthetic compounds is encountered rarely and may be suggested by a history of previous reactions. Measures to combat this eventuality must be available and instituted at once. The use of lidocaine or some other newer derivative may avoid sensitivity reactions. If a past history of reaction is obtained or suggested, it is wise to proceed cautiously; certainly, contact testing and small dilute solutions should be used first. With a definite history of sensitivity, other methods of treatment must be considered, especially in ambulatory patients.

When 10 ml or more of 1 per cent lidocaine is to be injected, it is wise to give the patient premedication with 1.5 grains (0.10 g) of sodium secobarbital or other quick-acting barbiturate 20 to 30 minutes in advance of the injection to counteract a possible adverse anesthetic reaction.

In case of accidental intravenous injection of a sizable amount of any of the "caines," or when symptoms of a definite hypersensitivity arise from any of these compounds, an ampoule of one of the soluble barbiturate preparations, such as sodium pentothal, should be introduced intravenously slowly according to the reaction and response. In addition oxygen should be administered through a clear airway (Bonica, 1953).

A depot corticoid given intravenously by chance has been reported (Murnaghan and McIntosh), but has not been observed by us. The manufacturers of each depot corticosteroid, in response to direct inquiries, state that no instance of accidental intravenous administration of their preparations has come to their attention.

Minor reaction from lidocaine and analgesic preparations consist of any of the following: slight dizziness, pallor, diaphoresis, weakness, nausea, rarely fainting and increased pulse rate. (A slowing of the pulse rate is a major symptom of reaction to intravenous adminstration.) The symptoms appear 5 to 15 minutes after injection as a rule, but they may be delayed for up to a few hours. Sometimes it is difficult to decide whether the reaction is due to hypersusceptibility or a vasomotor reaction to fright. The possibility of a reaction should be mentioned tactfully to the patient, so that it will be reported promptly to the physician. The patient should be allowed to remain in the office or clinic until any untoward symptoms disappear, and the pulse rate and blood pressure are normal.

Minor reactions are not contraindications. Some tense or hypersensitive individuals may be reactive in one way or another to any kind of needling. Such patients should be detected beforehand and given strong reassurance.

Every injection technique is subject to special anatomic hazards: (1) in the use of injections for periarticular structures and muscles, where a blood vessel may be entered in the line of approach under the skin; (2) in a locality where a cyst is to be aspirated, as in the popliteal space, in the vicinity of veins and arteries; (3) in injections of the chest or back, where deep penetration must be carried out with due regard for the underlying viscera. The most obvious precaution against entering a blood vessel is to aspirate after every one to 2 ml of solution injected. Penetration or flicking of a nerve may give sharp or lightning pain that disturbs the patient, and this possibility should be mentioned in advance.

The possibility of introducing infection is always a consideration in local injection. It is unlikely when local anesthetics alone are used, with careful, appropriate preparation of the site of injection. We have given thousands of such injections without once to our knowledge having caused this complication in any of our patients. When a corticosteroid is added to the anesthetic solution or injected alone deeply, it requires strict aseptic skin preparation. This will be described later.

Sometimes subcutaneous bleeding is produced by penetration of a fine venule, arteriole, or capillary in the course of giving an injection. We have not seen any serious consequence of such mishaps. The patient should be reassured that the discoloration or induration will be absorbed painlessly and advised to apply ice or cold compresses.

Rarely, after-pain lasting for several hours may follow injections. It may be due to the trauma from the needling, penetrating inflamed tissue, manipulation of a nerve, or indirect pressure on adjacent nerve tissue. The hyperemia following injection may give slight, transient discomfort. "After-pain" is usually relieved by local heat with an electric pad, hot-water bottle, or a warm soak followed by gentle massage; sometimes by local application of cold or ice.

SYSTEMIC EFFECTS

Unless some untoward reaction occurs, the temperature, sedimentation rate, blood count, and blood pressure are not influenced by analgesic therapy with anesthetic solution or with a small dose of corticosteroids.

INDICATIONS FOR ADDITION OF CORTICOSTEROIDS

Indications for addition of corticosteroids include the following:

1. A corticoid suspension may be added to an analgesic solution for local infiltration of tender soft tissue lesions when local response to the analgesic solution alone is short or inadequate. The combination yields good immediate comfort as well as the prolonged corticoid action for more effective local therapy.
2. Corticosteroids may be given for the relief of synovitis in tendon sheaths, bursae, or joints in inflammatory, noninfectious arthropathies, or for tenosynovial injection.
3. Most often corticosteroids are given as intraarticular therapy to suppress inflammation in one or two isolated, troublesome joints.
4. They provide adjunctive therapy for one or a few extremely resistant joints not responsive to other systemic therapy.
5. They control the most active joints when systemic corticosteroid administration is contraindicated.
6. They facilitate a rehabilitative and physical therapy program or orthopedic corrective procedures.
7. They are used to support a rheumatoid patient with active joint inflammation pending the effects of other systemic therapy (such as gold).

The prompt and gratifying relief derived from intraarticular therapy is a great boost to the patient's morale.

CONTRAINDICATIONS TO USE OF CORTICOSTEROIDS

Subsequent to intraarticular cortiscosteroids, some degree of systemic absorption ("spillover") may take place.

The usual precautions for steroid use apply especially to present or past peptic ulcer, diabetes mellitus, and infection. The accepted relative and absolute contraindications must be considered as for systemic therapy, especially if repeated injections are to be carried out.

Patients with uncontrolled diabetes are not desirable subjects for local corticoid injections. The severity of the complication compared with the urgency of the need for relief from musculoskeletal pain will determine the "relative" contraindication to such treatment.

When systemic or local infection is present or thromboembolic phenomena have developed, cortiscosteroid injections are contraindicated.

During anticoagulant therapy, needling of deep tissues is undesirable and may be hazardous. Even with injected corticoids, when given repeatedly in a series, rounding of the face or facial hirsutism may appear, but this recedes steadily after completion of treatment.

UNDESIRABLE REACTIONS

The most serious potential complication of the intraarticular administration of corticosteroids is the possible risk of introducing an infection. Although our extensive experience has shown that with scrupulous attention to asepsis this problem is avoided, the patient should be cautioned to immediately report development of the delayed onset of pain, redness or swelling at any recently injected joint. Thus, appropriate and effective treatment can be initiated promptly in the unlikely event that an infection has occurred. We do not recommend the routine prophylactic use of an antibiotic.

Other local adverse reactions are usually minor and reversible. Some localized subcutaneous or cutaneous atrophy resulting in a depigmented area of depression at the site of the injection may rarely develop, but usually resolves when the crystals of the steroid have been completely absorbed (Cassidy and Bole). Careful technique, avoiding the "tracking" or leaking of the steroid suspension into the dermis will prevent or minimize this complication.

The "post-injection flare" which may begin within a few hours after corticosteroid injection usually tends to subside spontaneously in several to 24 hours, rarely continuing up to 72 hours. In some instances, this may represent a true "crystal-induced synovitis" due to corticosteroid ester crystals (McCarty and Hogan). Usually the reaction is mild and adequately controlled with the application of ice and analgesics such as aspirin with codeine. The occurrence of a post-injection synovitis, sufficiently severe to require "reaspiration" of the joint to obtain relief is extremely rare.

LIMITATIONS

One of the chief characteristics of the therapeutic analgesic injection, whether it be a local injection or a nerve block, is the frequent need for repeated infiltration to obtain the desired result. Even in responsive conditions prolonged relief of pain may have to be maintained by two or more injections until results are adequate or lasting. Many times in suitable cases the repeated analgesia with "caine" compounds is not quite effective. The administration of corticosteroids alone or in combination with a "caine" then may be useful, usually at longer intervals.

DURATION OF ANALGESIA

Local and regional analgesic injection therapy has the advantage of permitting the application of effective medication at the site of irritation or pain, or at the source of nerve supply and pain radiation. Usually 30 minutes to 2 hours or more of local anesthesia follow. It is noteworthy that in many cases the analgesic effect continues after the anesthetic action disappears. In these cases, varying degrees of analgesia persist for one or several days, or even weeks or longer. The degree of benefit and its duration depend largely on (1) the underlying pathology, (2) the potential for response, (3) various personal characteristics of the patient, and (4) the pathophysiology. A placebo test may be informative and is desirable whenever practicable, preferably at the start of treatment in view of trigger areas appearing "in patterns of hysteria" (Travell and Bigelow).

PITFALLS AND OTHER CONSIDERATIONS

Lidocaine and its equivalent, or corticosteroid suspensions are, of course, not solvents for hypertrophic or degenerated tissue, or for any other pathologic lesions which may be the source of symptoms. Such injections must be used after due evaluation of the prospects of giving relief. These are judged by the cause and source of the symptoms and the stage of the pathology. Irreversible changes or disturbances in pathophysiology, systemic disease, and the patient's emotional status present difficulties in the use of analgesic injections unless such factors are recognized and the potential response evaluated in advance (Table 8).

Analgesic injections should not be regarded as a panacea to be used indiscriminately. In no case is analgesic block or infiltration justified without appropriate history and examination, and at least a tentative working diagnosis. Except perhaps in the severe acute discomfort of musculoskeletal origin that must be relieved at once, the usual therapeutic measures should first be given a fair trial. Indications, contraindications, and technique of injection must receive due attention. The results should be assessed with great care in emotional, apprehensive, and unstable individuals.

TABLE 8. Pitfalls in the Use of Analgesic Injections for Painful Musculoskeletal Disorders

1. Wrong diagnosis and incorrect localization of pain
2. Advanced pathology
   - irreversible changes
   - musculoskeletal inadequacy
3. Uncorrected contributory factors continuing trauma or strain (occupational or recreational)
   - poor body mechanics
     - bad posture, overweight, static defects (weak feet, bowlegs, knock-knees)
   - systemic factors
     - inflammation (rheumatoid and others), infections, angiopathy, focal infection, metabolic disorders (endocrine, diabetic, menopausal)
4. Multiple lesions, unrecognized
5. Refractoriness to “caine” drugs
6. Treatment of subjective complaints without objective findings
7. Hypersensitivity or low pain threshold
8. Overlooked skin hyperesthesia
9. Psychalgia
10. Lack of controls (e.g., lidocaine–saline–lidocaine test)

3

General Techniques for Local Injection of Soft Tissues

In Chapters 3 through 10 we will describe the application of local and regional anesthetic and analgesic procedures to the diagnosis and treatment of musculoskeletal pain. Only tried and safe methods are included —procedures that have been employed or observed repeatedly and frequently by the authors in the clinic, on the wards, or in private practice. When desirable, the source of technique is indicated. Highly specialized methods, such as facial and paravertebral nerve blocks, are not described because they require special training and are seldom indicated in everyday practice. General techniques are outlined in this chapter. Chapters 4 through 10 deal with injections in specific areas.

The materials and items required for local injection of soft tissues should be prepared and arranged in advance, to avoid time-consuming interruptions disturbing to the patient (see Table 5, page 7).

In preparing the site for injection for cleanliness and asepsis, we do the following:

For analgesic injections with lidocaine or equivalents, thorough cleansing of the skin with alcohol has proved adequate.

For the injection of corticosteroids we cleanse a generous area of skin with a detergent or cleanser, then use any of the standard antiseptics. A skin pencil first outlines the landmarks or situates the point of entry or the point of maximum tenderness (PMT). A cruciate or circular mark of broad lines can be drawn with tincture of iodine, a double layer applied with a sterile applicator. The wheal and then the entry are made at the center of a cross or circle. The iodine later is removed with alcohol. Aseptic handling of needles and syringes is imperative.

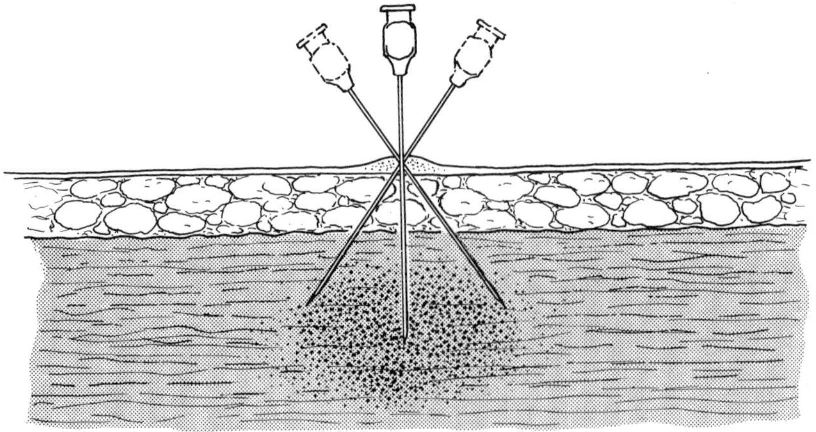

Fig. 3–1. Drawing (hypothetical) of a local tender point (subcutaneous induration or inflammation?).

INDICATIONS

Extensive observations have shown that local analgesic injection of any of the "caine" preparations, especially the newer ones, such as lidocaine, often is effective in suitable cases. Local injection at the palpable, most tender point is the simplest and most frequently used analgesic measure in traumatic and other forms of soft tissue involvement—myositis, myalgia, myofascitis, and in what is commonly called fibrositis (Fig. 3–1). Frequently affected sites are the connective tissues and muscles of the neck, shoulders, paraspinal, and gluteal areas, the regions about the fascias, such as the lumbodorsal fascia, as well as the connective tissue structures of the lumbosacral and sacroiliac areas in the low back; and inflammation or disturbances of any of the accessible "soft tissues."

Such disorders often are amenable to this method of treatment. Responsive tender points are located by palpation in and about the above structures. Other frequent sites are the large muscles of the neck, those over the scapulae, and those about the upper end of the humerus. In fact, tender points are frequent in the soft tissues at moving parts and about gliding surfaces (Fig. 3–2), as tabulated from a series of our own patients.

Basic principles discussed in this and other chapters must be applied for effective local analgesic injection (see Table 4, page 4).

LOCATING THE POINT OF MAXIMUM TENDERNESS

In addition to arriving at a diagnosis in painful disorders, the painful area is examined and the nature and site of maximum tenderness determined and evaluated by inspection, by manipulation, and by radiologic

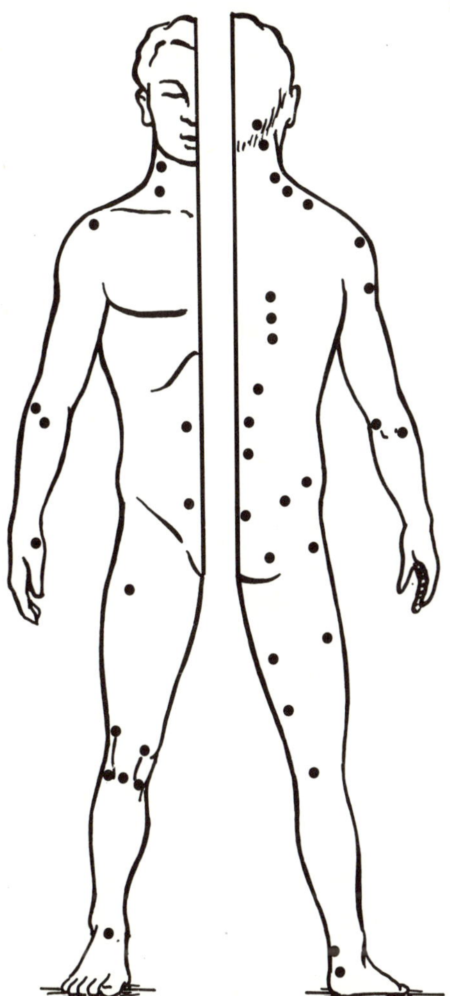

Fig. 3–2. The common point of maximum tenderness (PMT) in a series of sites. Note predominant locations at moving parts and sliding surfaces.

and other laboratory data. Localization by digital palpation provides the most significant findings. The examiner must try to identify and inject the actual source of pain in the affected tissues rather than in a zone of referred tenderness and pain radiation where relief is obtained simultaneously by infiltrating the true focal point (Fig. 3–3). In many cases a point of maximum tenderness can be localized (Steinbrocker 1941; Travell and Bigelow). The spot may be surrounded by a halo of lesser soreness, or areas of secondary discomfort may be palpated nearby. The point of greatest tenderness should be injected. There may be several such sites requiring infiltration before the symptoms are relieved. These should be

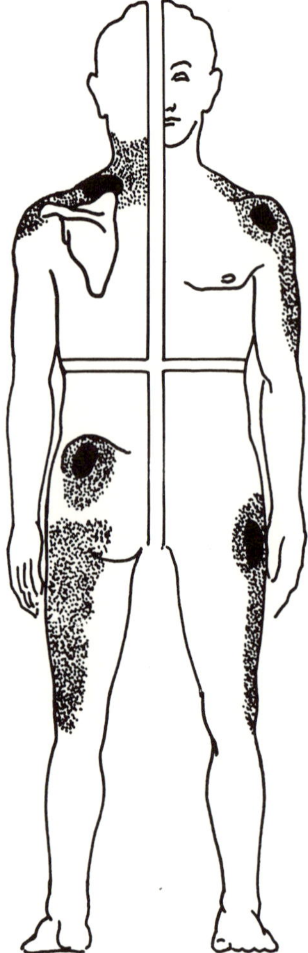

Fig. 3–3. Point of maximum tenderness (PMT), with surrounding satellite areas of lesser discomfort.

injected if they persist after effective infiltration of the point of maximum tenderness.

TECHNIQUE

Once the point or points of maximum soreness are determined and the site is prepared, each is marked with a superficial wheal. Now, with a 1- to 3-in. needle, 2.5 to 10 ml of aqueous lidocaine, or its equivalent, are injected through each wheal directly into the center of the painful site. The depth varies from 0.5 to 3 in., depending on the thickness of the subcutaneous tissues and musculature. When the structures to be injected lie over bone, e.g., over the scapula, it is safe to insert the needle boldly but gently straight down into the tissues (Fig. 3–1). If bone is touched, some solution is deposited and the needle is withdrawn slightly into the soft tissues where the rest of the medication is instilled.

A detailed description of all areas, especially muscles, likely to require local injection is not practical here. In general, when the structures to be infiltrated lie over soft, vulnerable parts, such as blood vessels or viscera, as in the chest or abdomen, especially careful technique is required. Examples are injections of the sternomastoid or trapezius muscles (*see* Chapter 4).

TENDER-POINT AND TRIGGER-POINT DISORDERS

Tender points, trigger points, and myalgic spots are terms used to describe circumscribed tenderness consistently demonstrable by palpation. These reflect special disturbances of the soft tissues—in and about muscles, in periarticular structures, and in various parts of the locomotor system. They differ from the many "algias" in presenting constant, reproducible points of maximum tenderness to palpation, whether or not migratory or intermittent muscular aches and pains are associated.

A "myalgic spot" or point of maximum tenderness in an area of pain or soreness more often is elicited in patients who complain of musculoskeletal pain—particularly muscular or periarticular—rather than a trigger point. To be responsive to therapy, however, the point of tenderness must show palpable soreness greater than any other soreness in the area of complaint, must be reproducible, and relieved within 5 to 10 minutes by an analgesic injection (Fig. 3–3).

A trigger point syndrome or disorder by definition exists when a sharply localized point of tenderness is evoked by palpation, and when pressure at that point reproduces the pain and radiation described by the patient; further, when the point is needled, the piercing reproduces the phenomena; and when injected with lidocaine solution, the symptoms are abolished with improved motion of the part. All of these requirements are not often fulfilled by disorders resembling trigger points. Induration may be felt by the pressing finger. More sensitized palpation of induration, bumps, and subcutaneous lumps is permitted by applying a lubricant, such as K-Y jelly, to the fingertips.

PRECAUTIONS

Each of the above disorders, for careful management, requires some precautions for control. It must be determined whether cutaneous hyperesthesia overlies the lesion and its distribution. The preliminary intracutaneous wheal alone at times may abolish the symptoms briefly or for some time. When practical, the lidocaine (wheal)-saline-lidocaine test should be carried out to assess the relative effectiveness of a neutral substance. This procedure starts with the lidocaine wheal. If palpation over the wheal still elicits soreness, 1-3 ml of normal saline is injected through the wheal subcutaneously or into the tender point in 15 minutes or at the next session; if relief is not obtained for an appreciable time, 1-5 ml of 1% lidocaine, depending on the depth and size of the sore spot, are injected. Should the saline produce a respectable response the final step is not necessary, or it may be carried out simply for information as to the patient's relative responsiveness.

The tender points and trigger points usually are localized in the musculature or in the juxtaarticular or periarticular soft tissues, often in or about the low back, neck, shoulders, paravertebral area, and gluteal muscles. The nodules felt by some observers, which they "rub out" or inject, may be points of circumscribed, local muscular spasm. Apart from the rheumatoid, lupoid, subcutaneous nodes encountered by us, we have not been successful in localizing such tender induration.

Tender points are apt to be felt at painful areas with extensive fibrous or connective tissues—large tendons, ligaments, or fascias—and also over periarticular structures and in the paravertebral regions. Soft tissues overlying moving parts are common sites. Frequently, nodulation with tenderness has been encountered by us at subcutaneous, fibrolipomatous deposits, usually with other nontender, palpable fatty nodules elsewhere. Theoretically, similar deep deposits with inflammatory or irritative reaction in components of fibrous tissue may account for the tender points in some subjects. Tendon sheaths under or adjacent to fibrolipomatous deposits may not be visibly swollen but the actual source of soreness. Herniation of fat lobules through fascia may be painful (Copeman and Ackerman).

The posterior superior spine of the pelvis is not infrequently the location of overlying, palpable induration, cyst-like or as a bursal node, without pain or tenderness. It may be unilateral or bilateral and insensitive. Sometimes these lesions become painful, tender, and enlarged. Occasionally, similar, palpable and uncomfortable developments are encountered at the ischial tuberosity. These may become troublesome in rheumatoid arthritis (Françon).

SIMPLE LOCAL TECHNIQUES

Ethyl chloride or any other vapocoolant spray for light freezing of the skin (without frosting) at and about tender areas may be helpful by itself, without injections in some cases, especially when repeated at home as needed several times during the day or at longer intervals in 10 to 15 passes over the tender area. (The flammability of the spray as well as the undersirability of inhaling the anesthetic are major drawbacks of this form of therapy.)

In patients who are hypersensitive to both a needled skin wheal or freezing with ethyl chloride, we have, with the patient's consent, used the "cold turkey" injection—a quick jab through the skin. A helpful method of skin anesthesia now used for such individuals is the mechanical intracutaneous spray wheal with the Dermo-Jet instrument discussed in Chapter 1. The Hypospray, a larger device, may serve well for the whole procedure. These instruments make treatment by injection more acceptable to patients who are hypersensitive to or fearful of needling.

TRAUMATIC LESIONS

Simple local injuries usually heal spontaneously with little, if any, medical care. When severe pain is presented, traumatic disorders not infrequently can be relieved and functional recovery expedited by the immediate analgesic infiltration of sprains and contusions. The demonstrated value of the procedure in a variety of painful, traumatic conditions will not be considered here. Careful examination and X-ray films always are in order to exclude fracture or dislocation. More rapid relief of pain and disability has been observed in acute conditions when the patients are treated within 24 hours after injury.

The methods described for localized soft tissue lesions, fibrositis, or periarthritis, may be employed. Daily or less frequent injection may be required for severe symptoms, usually one to three treatments sufficing. Increased pain may follow injection, but it wears off soon. When chronic disorders are present, prolonged therapy may become necessary. The blocks should then supplement physical therapy and massage, if the latter have proved inadequate.

Muscular contusions are a form of traumatic soft tissue lesion or traumatic fibrositis. They may arise in any of the superficial or deep muscles, especially in the region of the neck, the trapezius, and deltoid muscles, the muscles of the forearms, the low back, and the flexors and extensors of the legs; they may be treated effectively by analgesic infiltration. When traumatic disorders are intractable to such treatment, orthopedic consultation is indicated. Analgesic methods are useful in markedly painful situations, or in conditions unresponsive to simpler measures.

The role of "somatic trigger areas in the patterns of hysteria" (Travell and Bigelow) often requires evaluation.

The dangers of using analgesic injections must be considered (see Table 8, page 22).

PRINCIPLES OF LOCAL TECHNIQUES

1. The more sharply and consistently demarcated the point of maximum tenderness, the more likely its response to local injection therapy.
2. Effective use of local injections (with lidocaine, corticosteroid suspension, or both) is demonstrated by increasing intervals of relief.
3. Use of analgesic solutions (lidocaine or equivalent) is simpler and should be evaluated first, if practical, before introducing cortiscosteroids.
4. The lidocaine-saline-lidocaine test provides helpful information concerning placebo-reactors and the correct localization of the source of pain.
5. The behavior of the needle-shy patient and his reaction to injected medication must be considered before and after any procedure.
6. The sharply circumscribed point of tenderness responsive to analgesic solution, if only for the duration of anesthesia, is apt to respond beneficially to repeated injections of lidocaine solution alone or to added corticosteroid suspension at increasing intervals.

4

The Head Region

OCCIPITAL NERVE BLOCK

Occipital neuritis or neuralgia may be presented by rheumatic patients. A point of maximum tenderness usually can be localized over the greater occipital nerve as it passes over the external occipital protuberance. This must be distinguished from localized or diffuse tenderness in the extensive connective tissue of the cervicooccipital area.

TECHNIQUE FOR GREATER OCCIPITAL NERVE BLOCK

The greater occipital nerve originates at the posterior division of the second cervical nerve. The site of injection is a point just above the superior nuchal line, about 1 in. from the midline. Palpation of the occipital artery lateral to the nerve serves as a further guide. An adequate patch of scalp should be shaved to ensure a clean, sterile injection (Fig. 4–1).

A hypodermic needle is used and its entry along the line of the occipital nerve should produce paresthesias that indicate correct placement. Three to 5 ml or 0.5 to 1.0 per cent lidocaine are used at 3- to 7-day intervals or longer.

TECHNIQUE FOR OCCIPITAL OR CERVICOOCCIPITAL TENDER POINTS

Sometimes circumscribed sore points are palpated at the hairline or in the tissues of the suboccipital area.

Neuritic or neuralgic tenderness not infrequently is associated with symptoms of postural strain, fibrositis, or degenerative cervical spondylosis. Diffuse tenderness often is found, but trigger points may be localized

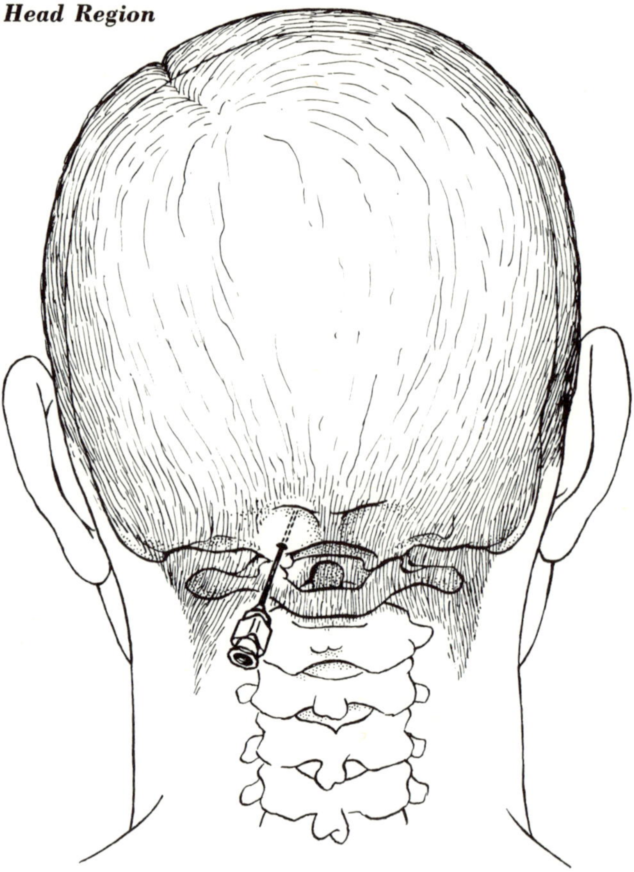

Fig. 4–1. Greater occipital nerve block.

in this area. They usually are accessible and responsive to infiltration. Good localization of tenderness in the soft tissue of this region leads to effective infiltration of the points of tenderness whether superficial or deep.

Most often the maximum tender point is at one or both sides of the midline 1.0 to 2.0 cm from it in the soft tissues of the infraoccipital area. Injection of these circumscribed tender points with 1 to 3 ml of lidocaine frequently is effective (Fig. 4–2). It is possible and convenient to enter just below the hairline and reach the point of tenderness or the occipital border by directing the needle upward. One or more further infiltrations at intervals of 3 to 7 or more days may be needed.

Paravertebral block of the cervical nerves or infiltration of the brachial plexus may relieve radicular pain or deep tissue discomfort in the cervical area that is not responsive to local injections. Cervical neuralgia or os-

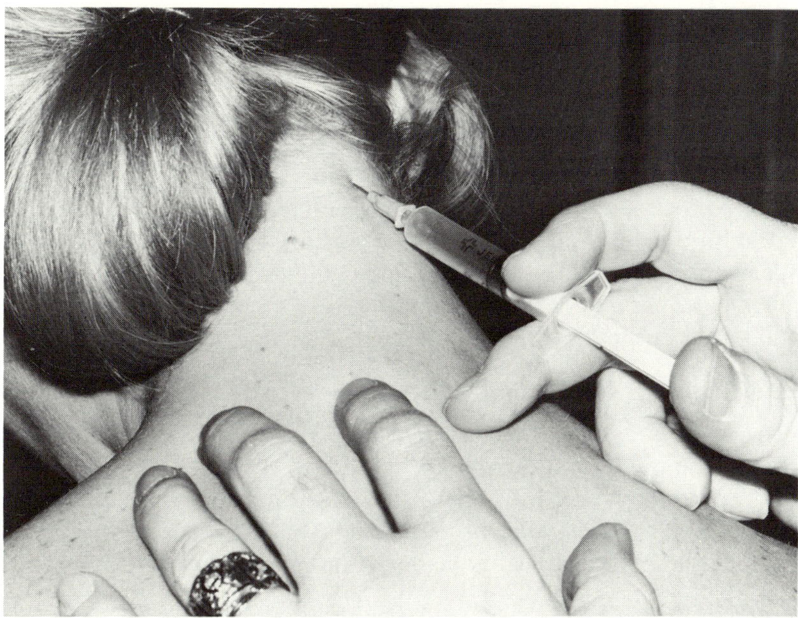

Fig. 4–2. Injection of point of maximum tenderness (PMT) in suboccipital area.

teoarthrosis of the cervical spine with neural symptoms also may be treated by this method, when associated with localized tenderness.

Sympathetic Stellate Ganglion Block

Sympathetic cervical ganglion block, usually of the stellate ganglion, is indicated occasionally for postherpetic neuralgia of the face, neck, shoulder region, or upper limb, for early reflex dystrophy, and particularly in the early shoulder-hand syndrome. Like paravertebral cervical block, this method may provide effective relief in special, intractable situations.

The procedure requires special technique (page 49).

INJECTION OF TEMPOROMANDIBULAR JOINT

INDICATIONS

The temporomandibular joint may require articular or periarticular injection because of pain or troublesome trismus. Discomfort and dysfunction may accompany nonspecific involvement of the facial muscles, mechanical disorders about the temporomandibular joint, degenerative changes, and rheumatoid or other inflammatory articular involvement localizing at one or both joints. A dental, and sometimes an otorhinologic, evaluation may be helpful.

TECHNIQUE

The patient lies supinely with the head facing upward, or sits in a chair with the head supported. The zygomatic arch is palpated with the ends of the fingers. The tip of the index finger is placed inferior to the arch about 2 cm anterior to the tragus of the ear. When the patient opens and closes her mouth, the condyle of the ascending ramus is felt.

Periarticular or Intraarticular Injection

The point of entry lies just inferior to the zygomatic arch and halfway between the tragus and the anterior border of the ascending ramus (Fig. 4–3). The pulsation of the superficial temporal artery is palpated somewhat posterior to this point near the tragus of the ear with the patient's mouth closed. A skin wheal is made at the point selected, approximately

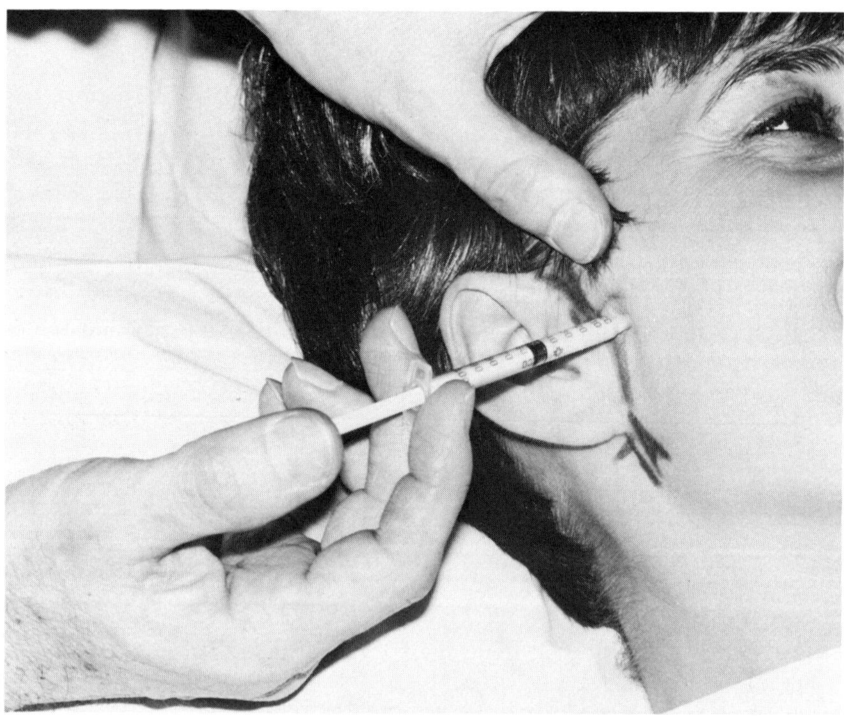

Fig. 4–3. Temporomandibular injection.

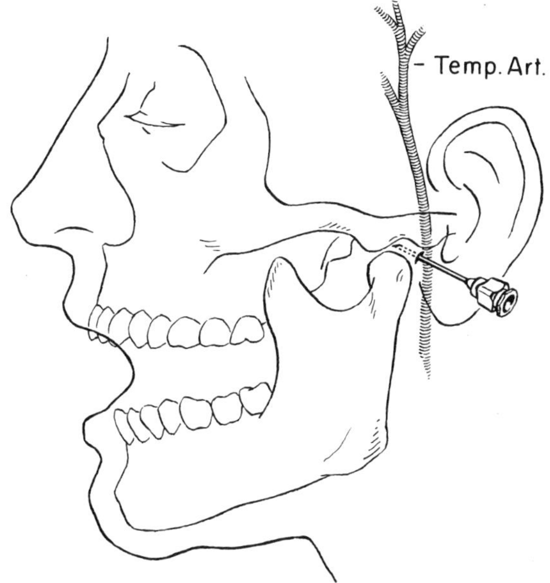

Fig. 4–4. Intraarticular temporomandibular injection.

one fingerbreadth anterior to the ear. A 1- or 1.5-in., 22-G needle is then inserted through the wheal perpendicular to the surface of the skin. The ramus is near the surface, almost subcutaneous. When bone is touched, 2 or 3 ml of lidocaine solution are deposited for a periarticular infiltration. Aspiration before injection is advisable.

The procedure may be done intraarticularly after the needle rests on the condyle by having the patient open the mouth (Fig. 4–4). Then the needle is slipped from the condyle up 0.15 cm or less into the joint. Aspiration is done and the injection is given. It may be repeated at intervals of 5 to 7 days until adequate relief is obtained. Usually, it is not necessary to give more than one to three injections. If inflammation is suspected, or if the patient has rheumatoid disease, a corticosteroid suspension, such as 10 mg of prednisolone TBA, is added to the intraarticular injection and longer intervals allowed. If no increasing benefit follows one or two sessions, the procedure should be terminated and other causes or remedies considered.

INJECTION OF THE NECK REGION

Pain, tenderness, and spasticity of muscles in the region of the neck, especially the sternomastoid, trapezius, erector spinae and deltoid muscles, frequently occur in the various systemic rheumatologic diseases and in nonspecific soft tissue disorders. If such symptoms do not respond to ordinary measures, and there is circumscribed tenderness to palpation, local injection therapy may control the complaints.

STERNOMASTOID MUSCLE INJECTION

The sternomastoid muscle is injected after the point of maximum tenderness is localized. The patient is treated with the head turned slightly toward the affected side so as to relax the muscle. Over the point of maximum tenderness, along the line of the muscle, a skin wheal is made. The tender surrounding muscle is grasped between the thumb and forefinger and raised slightly. The injection is made through the wheal into the muscle mass (Fig. 4–5). The dose is 3 to 5 ml of 0.5 to 1.0 per cent lidocaine solution or its equivalent.

Any other muscle of the neck that yields a point of maximum tenderness to palpation after localizing the circumscribed tender points may

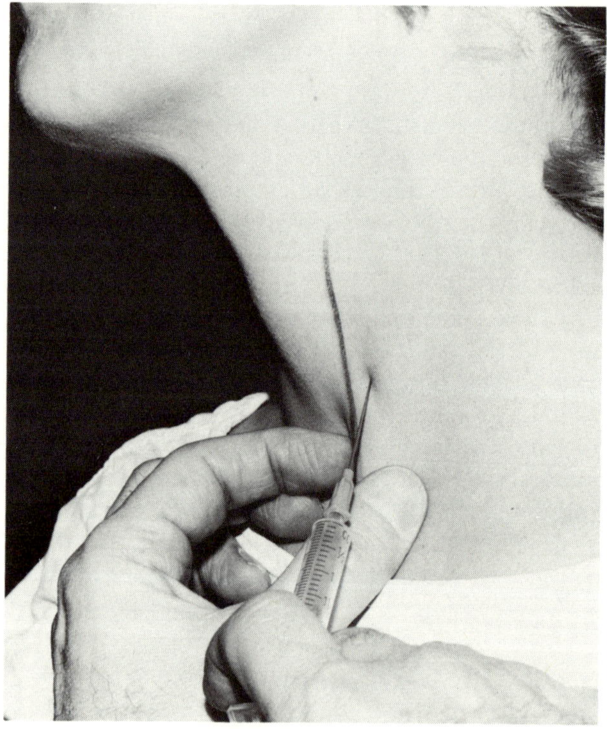

Fig. 4–5. Injection of sternomastoid muscle. The muscle belly about the tender point is brought up for insertion of the needle.

be infiltrated similarly. The determination and evaluation of overlying cutaneous hyperesthesia is helpful in this area.

The supraspinatus muscle often is injected (Fig. 9). The underlying scapula is readily touched with the tip of the needle, which then is withdrawn slightly for the injection.

SCALENUS ANTICUS BLOCK

The scalenus anticus block has value for diagnosis and treatment of cervicobrachial symptoms arising from thoracic outlet disorders. Neuralgic and neurovascular symptoms due to compression of brachial nerves by the scalenus anticus muscle should be relieved for at least 1 to 2 hours by the scalenus block. It is a particular consideration in the neuralgias associated with the thoracic outlet syndrome arising from scalenus anticus pressure, either primary or secondary.

The technique of injection (Gage) is a delicate procedure. The patient assumes the recumbent position, with the head turned toward the unaffected side. The scalenus anticus muscle is palpated posterior and lateral to the sternomastoid muscle. While the index finger of the left hand palpates the lateral border of the scalenus muscle, a 0.375-in. 25-G needle is inserted into its lateral edge through a skin wheal. The muscle is then infiltrated with 1 per cent lidocaine through its lower half, care being taken not to perforate it and thereby infiltrate elements of the brachial plexus or sympathetic nerve supply (Fig. 4-6). Within 5 to 10 minutes the scalenus anticus should be completely relaxed and the patient

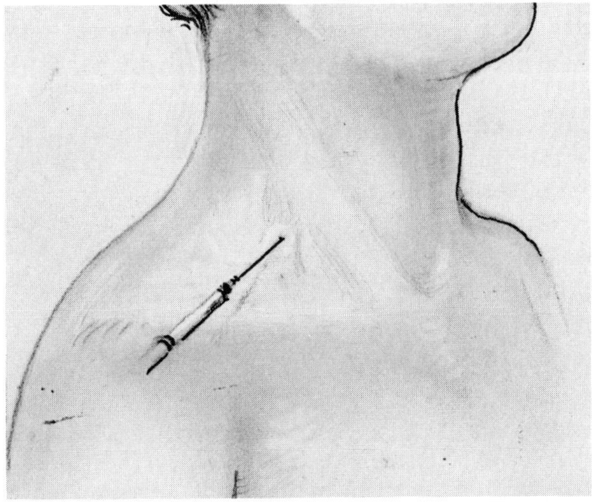

Fig. 4–6. Scalenus anticus muscle block (courtesy of Dr. Mims Gage).

temporarily relieved of the symptoms. Repeating the procedure in a few days may provide added relief, or a brief response may be seen as an indication for further evaluation, before surgical consideration.

PARAVERTEBRAL TENDER POINTS IN THE NECK REGION

Torticollis, "cricks," soreness, and stiffness of the neck muscles may be common, fleeting symptoms, but pain and stiffness sometimes may become prolonged, especially in the lateral and posterior musculature. The point of maximum tenderness may be found by palpation at any of the muscles of the neck, but frequently at the sternomastoid, trapezius, supra- or infraspinatus sites, or in the paravertebral area. The neck muscles are especially sensitive to drafts, trauma, and vertebral instability. Cervical osteoarthrosis often is associated with symptoms of the neck and cervicothoracic area. Tension and muscular fatigue occur frequently and may be contributory. The usual preventive measures are in order.

Technique

When tenderness is localized consistently by palpation, generally at lateral or posterior structures, associated with pain unresponsive to other measures, local injection is in order. If the condition is in an early stage, an analgesic injection of 2 to 5 ml of 0.5% lidocaine is used, with due care for any vulnerable anatomical structures. At the neck, special caution is necessary to avoid vascular or pulmonary (apical) penetration (Figs. 4–5 and 4–6).

When an injection is given posteriorly within 1 in. of the midline, any hazards from entering vascular or visceral structures in the neck are unlikely, especially if aspiration is carried out before the injection. The needle should not penetrate more than 0.75 to 1.0 in. Further probing is likely to touch the mass of the body or transverse process of a vertebra; then the needle is drawn back $\frac{1}{16}$ in. or more prior to injection.

Paravertebral cervical nerve block may be a useful technique for the persistent pain of cervical osteoarthrosis, the disc syndrome, or radiculitis in subjects unresponsive to other measures and unsuitable for surgery. It requires special technique.

5

The Shoulder Region

Analgesic injections of the painful shoulder may be accomplished by the following methods:

1. Local injection of the subcutaneous tissue, periarticular muscles, tendons, bursae, or shoulder cuff at the site of maximum tenderness, or at the presumed source of symptoms.
2. Aspiration of the shoulder joint and intraarticular injection.
3. Capsular and rotator cuff injection (adhesive capsulitis).
4. Sympathetic (stellate ganglion) injection.
5. Suprascapular nerve block.
6. Brachial plexus block.
7. Cervicodorsal (paravertebral) block of individual nerves.

The first three approaches are routine procedures. The others require special skills. Local injections will be discussed first, and then the special techniques used for intrinsic disorders of the shoulder.

LOCAL INJECTION

Local injections consist of infiltrating points of tenderness in the soft tissues about the shoulder area and at muscular sites of involvement accessible to palpation, such as the scapular and parascapular region, the deltoid, the paravertebral musculature and other soft tissues. The infiltration of tender points and trigger points in muscular or other soft tissues in this area follows the principles discussed above.

Local injections are administered subcutaneously, usually intramuscularly, or into the supportive tissue, at a level which is estimated from the amount of pressure required to evoke tenderness. Periarticular, paravertebral, and other soft tissue involvement often responds to these analgesic injections. In situations not adequately relieved, a corticosteroid may be added to the analgesic solution—10 to 20 mg of prednisolone suspension, or its equivalent.

TECHNIQUE

The point of maximum tenderness may be located at one or more sites consistent with any of the specific anatomical involvements already mentioned. Through a skin wheal over the tender point 1 to 5 ml of 1% lidocaine is instilled (Fig. 5-1).

INTRINSIC DISORDERS

Lesions of the supraspinatus tendon are a more frequent source of symptoms at the shoulder than all others combined. The condition may be acute, subacute, or chronically painful. It may recur sooner or later, even after the most gratifying response.

The supraspinatus tendon lying under the subdeltoid bursa is apt to

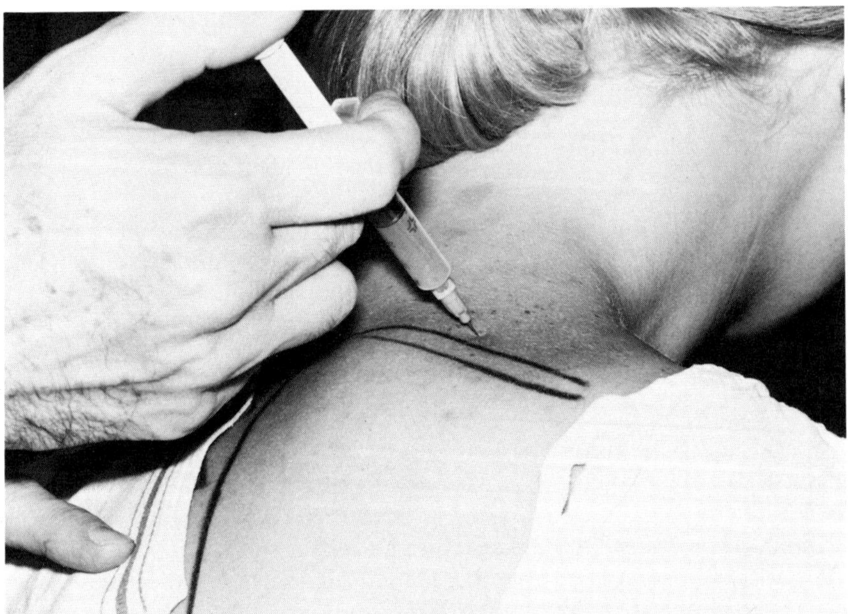

Fig. 5–1. Injection of tender point in the supraspinatus muscle.

produce adjacent bursitis when sufficient calcific, inflammatory provocation exists and spreads to the overlying bursal tissue. The bursitis is secondary and often accompanies the tenosynovitis, sometimes in florid form with effusion.

Acute and hyperacute symptoms, when the patient is in such extreme pain as to beg the physician not to touch the extremity, are usually present after one or more nights of disturbed sleep. The limbs of such patients should be moved as little as possible during the examination, and injections should be given with the patient supine. Premedication and thorough, gentle, local infiltration of anesthetic solution are helpful precautions. Treatment of the shoulder, after a preliminary hypodermic of meperidine, in the emergency room of the hospital, where the patient can rest a while, is the most desirable method in hyperacutely painful shoulder disability.

Subacute and chronic, intermittent or continued symptoms may occur. The treatment is the same with less likelihood of the degree and speed of response seen in the acute.

ASPIRATION AND INJECTION OF ACUTE CALCIFIC (SUPRASPINATUS) TENOSYNOVITIS (BURSITIS)

Technique

The injection is given at the point of maximum tenderness, usually below the acromion. When the tenderness is diffuse or not adequately localized, a point is chosen over the hiatus palpable between the anterolateral or anteromedial portion of the acromial border and the head of the humerus (Figs. 5–2A and 5–3).

The patient sits up with the extremity resting on the lap. After preparing the site, a skin wheal is made with lidocaine 1%. A 2-in., 22-G needle is attached to a 10-ml syringe (containing 1 ml of lidocaine for anesthetizing its track). The needle is directed perpendicularly to the skin surface, or pointing upward at an angle of 10 degrees, to penetrate the wheal and pass through the hiatus under the acromion. After penetrating 0.75 to 1.25 in., aspiration is carried out for fluid and calcific material (Figs. 5–2A and 5–3). The syringe is then removed, leaving the needle in place. Another syringe containing 1 ml of lidocaine with 25 to 50 mg of prednisolone suspension or its equivalent is attached and the medication is injected.

This procedure often is carried out only once, but it may have to be repeated once or twice in acute disorders. The calcium may disappear thereafter. It does so spontaneously, not infrequently, after any type of needling, or without it.

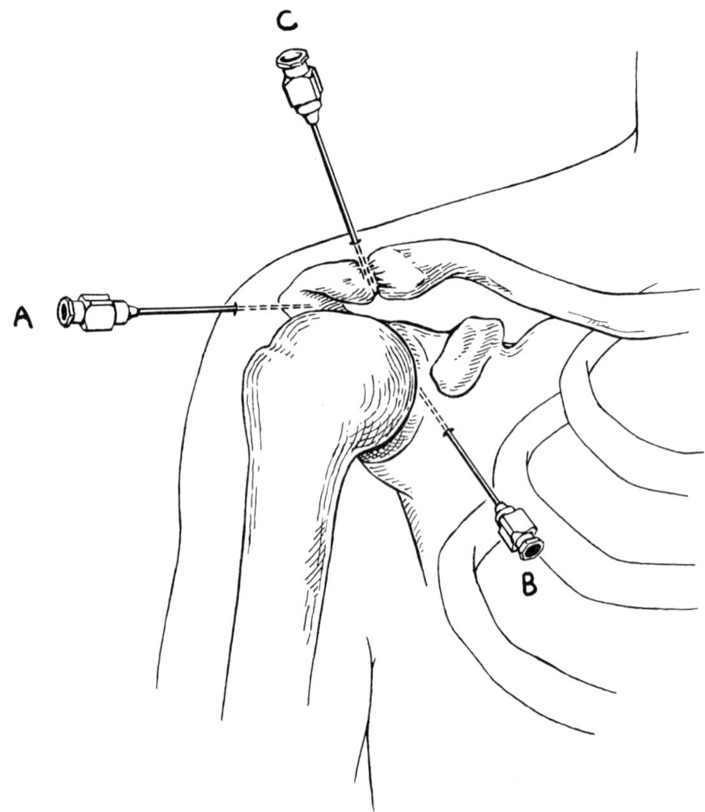

Fig. 5–2. *A.* Injection of subacromial bursa or at the supraspinatus tendon. *B.* Anterior approach for aspiration and injection of the scapulohumeral joint. *C.* Injection of the acromioclavicular joint.

In subacute or chronic calcific disorders with pain, and certainly with any degree of disability, one or two of these injections are worth a trial. If there is no apparent improvement, indicated by longer intervals of comfort, other approaches must be considered.

The location of the calcific deposit in the X-ray films is a useful guide. Sometimes the calcific material is somewhat inferior to the usual point of entry for calcification of the supraspinatus tendon. In that case, after penetrating the wheal, the needling is directed downward to the calcareous deposit, aspiration is tried, and a good portion of the medication is deposited there. The needle is then redirected to complete infiltration in the usual manner.

In any of these entries, if the needle happens to pierce inflamed tissue, a painful and sometimes severe reaction may follow when the analgesic

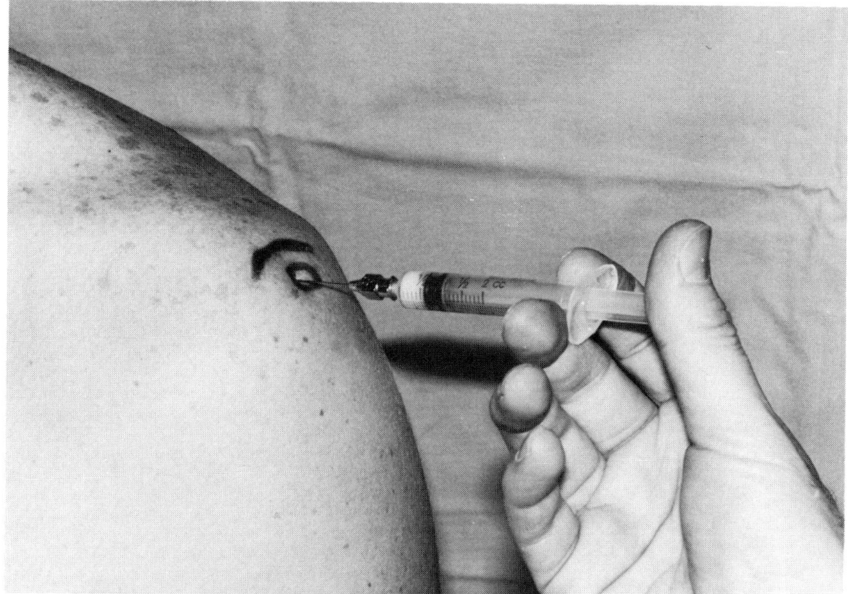

Fig. 5–3. Subacromial injection.

has worn off. To avoid undue concern, the patient should be cautioned about this possibility and should be instructed as to medication to take in such an eventuality.

Acute subdeltoid (or subacromial) bursitis may occur with swelling and visible or palpable fluctuation of the bursa, generally as a complication of rheumatoid arthritis or an adjacent tenosynovitis. In this case, the most palpable and fluctuant prominence may be used as a point of entry for aspiration of fluid and the injection of medication.

If the X-ray films show a fair amount of accessible calcific material, and the patient is not in too great pain, a large gauge, 2-in. needle, such as 16 to 18 G, may be used in an effort to aspirate the calcific deposit by multiple exploratory punctures in different directions after entry, followed by instillation of the lidocaine-corticoid combination. It is wise to prepare such a patient with an adequate amount of premedication with codeine or meperidine; this is perhaps most comfortably accomplished in the emergency room or during an overnight stay in the hospital.

If the above approaches are not feasible, the patient should be given an analgesic perorally, such as 30 mg of codeine, provided arrangements are made for someone to accompany the patient to her home. Then, in the supine position, after a skin wheal and with subcutaneous introduction of 1 per cent lidocaine as the needle travels, a subacromial supra-

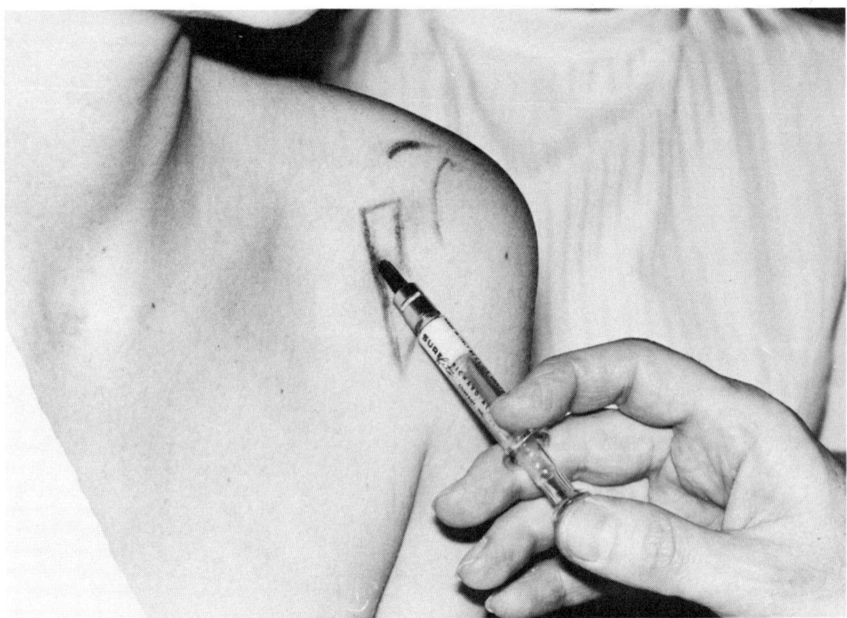

Fig. 5–4. Bicipital tendinous or peritendinous injection; with the patient seated, the arm is externally rotated.

spinatus infiltration of combined lidocaine (1 ml) and prednisolone (25 mg) suspension is given (Fig. 5–2A). No effort is made to probe for the tendon or to needle the bursa. The material is then deposited with suitable dispatch.

Bicipital tenosynovitis is frequently the source of symptoms in the painful shoulder in acute, subacute, or chronic form. In addition to palpable tenderness or "rolling" of the tendon, a confirmatory Yergason's test is a good diagnostic aid. This test elicits pain felt along the long head of the tendon when the hand of that side, grasping the examiner's, is externally rotated (supinated) against the examiner's resistance. The opposite hand of the examiner holds the patient's elbow to her side as the maneuver is carried out. A Speed test with the examiner resisting elevation of the extended upper limb as it is raised also is helpful, producing pain in the line of the bicipital tendon when positive.

Technique. The bicipital tendon and the borders of its groove are almost always palpable and any special tenderness can be determined. The tendon usually can be rolled with the examiner's fingertip. The opposite (asymptomatic) side is tested as a control and as an index of the patient's sensitivity.

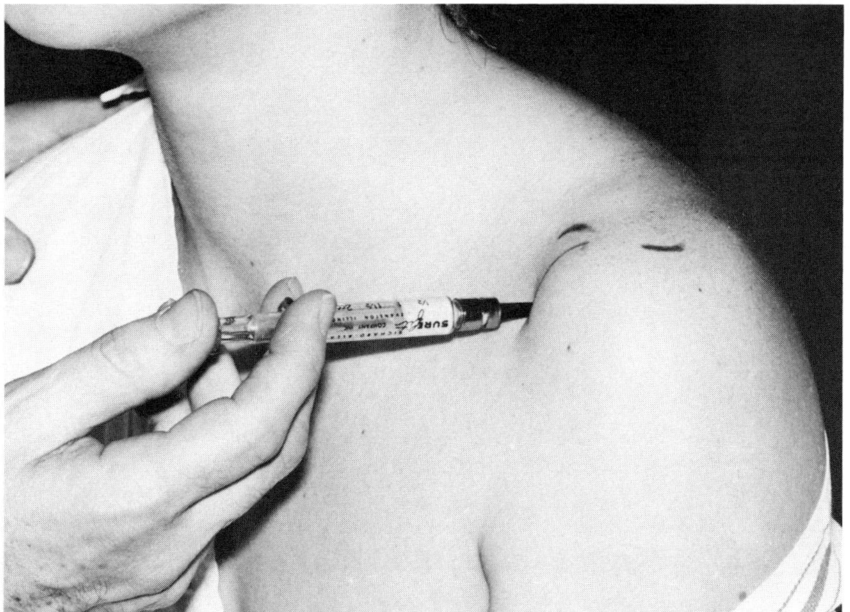

Fig. 5–5. The anterior approach to the shoulder joint.

At the midpoint of the line of tenderness, the entry is made through a skin wheal (Fig. 5–4). The needle is brought in along the side of the tendon aimed at one border of the bicipital groove to give a peritendinous infiltration (Fig. 5–5). One-third of the injection is given at this point. The needle is then withdrawn slightly, but kept subcutaneous, redirected upward about an inch for another one-third of the injection, withdrawn again and redirected downward, touching the bicipital border gently and the remainder deposited (Fig. 5–6). A series of injections of lidocaine (3 to 5 ml), alone or with prednisolone (25 mg), often is required.

A tear of the long head of the biceps or of other muscle fibers may occur. This may be associated immediately or later with circumscribed pain and tenderness. When a partial or complete rupture of the long head of the biceps is recent, it should be decided, with orthopedic consultation, whether surgical intervention is indicated. With long-standing pain and localized tenderness, simple measures may suffice.

ACUTE SCAPULOHUMERAL SYNOVITIS

When there is noticeable effusion into the shoulder joint the point of bulging or greatest tenderness is the best point of entry for aspiration

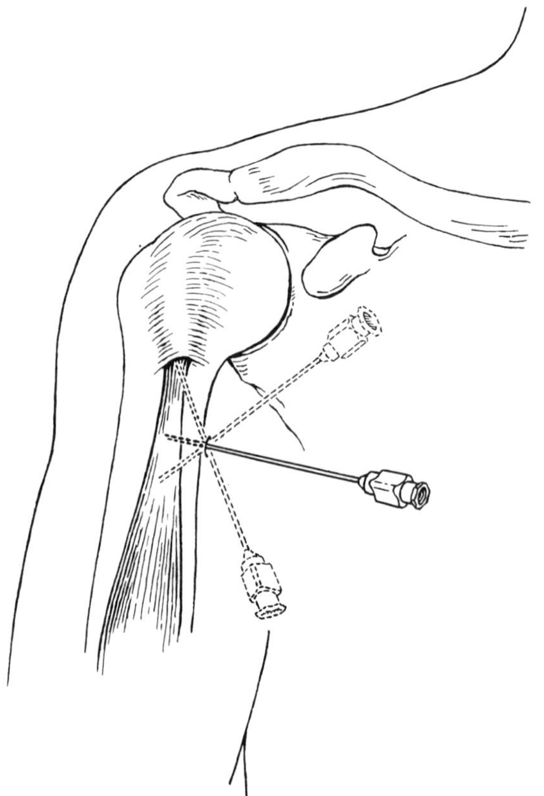

Fig. 5–6. The fanwise method of injection of or at the bicipital tendon.

and intracapsular or intraarticular injection, usually at the anterior or anteromedial aspect. Otherwise, the standard entry into the capsule or joint space is made by the anterior or posterior route.

Anterior Aspiration and Intraarticular Injection

Entry is made through a cutaneous wheal at a point medial to the head of the humerus and below the palpable tip of the coracoid process (Fig. 5–2*B*). A 2-in., 20- or 22-G needle is directed mediodorsally to the scapulohumeral interspace for about 0.75 in.; after aspiration of any fluid, 2 ml of lidocaine with 25 mg of prednisolone suspension are introduced through the same needle.

The posterior approach is practicable because it is done out of the patient's line of vision (Figs. 5–7 and 5–8). Internal rotation and adduction of the patient's arm, with the hand placed on the opposite shoulder and the elbow resting against the chest wall may be helpful. This opens the joint space and tightens the capsule, thus aiding penetration by the

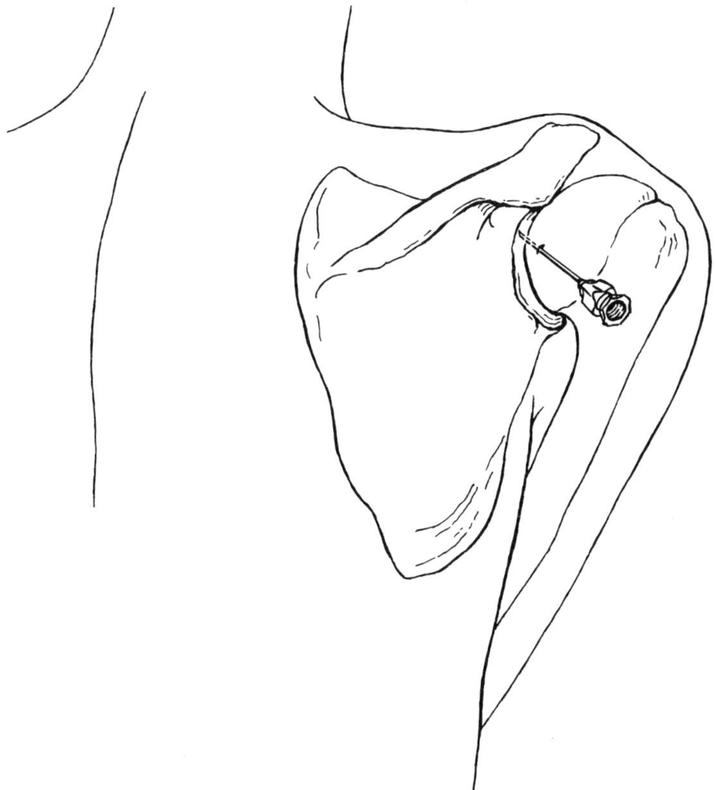

Fig. 5–7. Posterior approach to the capsule of the shoulder.

needle. A wheal is made at a point 0.75 to 1 in., depending on the size of the patient, from the posterolateral angle of the acromion, just under its posteroinferior border. A 2-in. 20- or 22-G needle is introduced through the wheal anteromedially to a point visualized as the capsule of the scapulohumeral articulation (1.0 to 1.5 in.). The needle seems to penetrate a free space. Aspiration and intracapsular injection are then carried out.

SCAPULOHUMERAL CAPSULITIS

Scapulohumeral capsulitis (frozen shoulder, periarthritis of the shoulder, adhesive capsulitis) may be acute, subacute, or chronic, and may be secondary to, or associated with, trauma and other pathology in the cervical area or spine. Most frequently it is seen as the idiopathic frozen shoulder. It often resolves spontaneously in 6–24 months or longer with an initial 2–4 months of pain, but disability throughout. Residual limita-

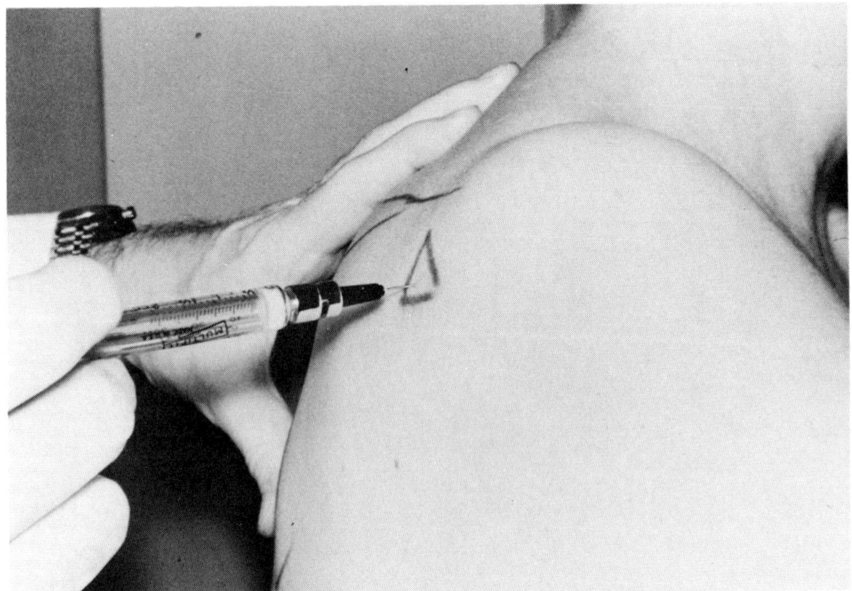

Fig. 5–8. Posterior approach to the shoulder.

tion remains in a small number of patients. In our hands it responds to injection treatment in over 85% of cases, with good to complete recovery of function (75 to 100% mobility) within 3 to 8 sessions. (Steinbrocker *et al.*) In a small percentage of cases as many as 10 or more sessions may be required. We follow a variation of the method of Crisp and Kendall. Three sites are infiltrated in rotation, and two of the three at each treatment session. They are (1) the supraspinatus tendon at the subacromial area; (2) the bicipital tendon by the fanwise method described above; and (3) the intracapsular injection of the shoulder joint by the anterior or posterior route.

The standard dosage and techniques are employed for each of these procedures. Naturally, when giving a corticosteroid, one must calculate the total amount of the compound that is administered at each visit and during a period of time. These treatments are given every 3 to 4 days during the first 7 to 10 days until the "hot" period of pain at the shoulder, especially nocturnal pain, subsides. Ordinarily, when first seen the disorder has been troublesome for at least 2 to 4 months. The suppression of pain during rest or motion proceeds steadily within the first 2 weeks, when this method is effective. Nocturnal pain usually disappears after 2 or 3 sessions; then treatments are given weekly and at progressively longer intervals.

A routine of graded shoulder exercises is indicated when nocturnal pain has been abolished. Tenderness at any site about the shoulder may persist for some time after pain has resolved and motion is restored. It disappears spontaneously after treatment is completed. Injections are discontinued when the patient shows 75 to 85% recovery of mobility as well as abolition of pain. Thereafter, we have found, natural mobilization of the residual limitation takes place without additional injections, completely in 80 to 90% of patients, and adequately in the remainder. Daily exercises are continued for approximately 3 months, but strenuous use of the arm should be avoided for 6 months.

STELLATE GANGLION BLOCK

This procedure is used in early shoulder-hand syndrome and painful reflex dystrophy of the upper extremity, in vasospastic disorders, in hyperhidrosis of the hands, and in reflex vasospasm of vascular injury, among other disorders.

Infiltration of the ganglion permits interruption of sympathetic nerve impulses through the cervicothoracic chain. The anterior (paratracheal) method of Finley and Patzer, as modified by Smith, is used.

Technique

The patient is placed in the supine position with the face directed upward (Figs. 5–9 and 5–10). The chin is elevated slightly. The injector stands at the side. The middle and index fingers of the left hand are placed about 1 to 2 cm apart along the medial border of the sternomastoid muscle, with the lower finger just above and against the sternoclavicular joint. The fingertips are pressed down slowly but firmly into the neck. The carotid pulsation is felt on the volar surface of the fingers. The dome of the lung, occasionally rising into the neck, is then displaced downward and the transverse processes and side of the bodies of the lower cervical vertebrae are felt by the fingertips.

"All important structures are displaced in this way and the stellate ganglion in its position against the underlying bony surface of the body and base of the transverse process of the seventh cervical vertebra is brought into a subcutaneous position between the examining fingers where it can be infiltrated safely" (Smith).

Ten ml of 1 per cent lidocaine is used for the injection, without epinephrine, via a 2-in. 22-G needle. The needle is inserted 2 fingerbreadths directly above the sternoclavicular joint perpendicularly through the skin surface adjacent to the trachea, down to the area of the ganglion. The bony surface of the transverse process indicates the area. If it is not touched, the soft ligamentous tissue between the processes or the inter-

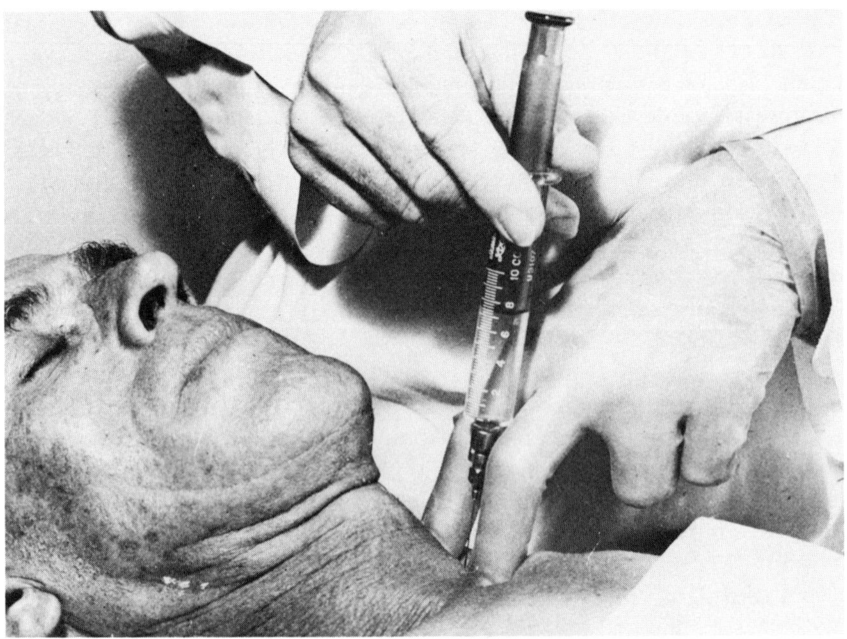

Fig. 5–9. Anterior stellate ganglion block. (From Smith, DW. *Amer J Surg* 82: 344, 1951.)

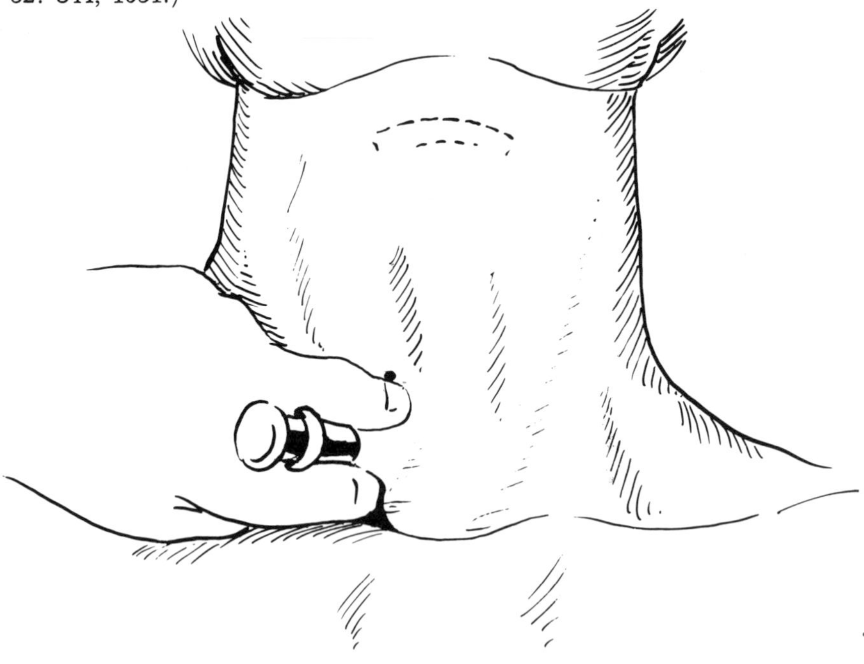

Fig. 5–10. Anterior stellate ganglion block showing fingers and needle in position. (From Smith, DW. *Amer J Surg* 82: 344, 1951.)

vertebral cartilage may be recognized, and the needle is then directed to a slightly higher or lower level. The solution is injected with frequent interruptions for aspiration.

Horner's syndrome (miosis, ptosis of the upper lid with narrowing of the palpebral fissure and congestion of sclera) appearing within a few minutes signals a successful nerve block. Within 10 to 20 minutes, warmth and dryness of the hand, forearm and side of the face may be noted and some visible flushing observed.

The procedure may be repeated a few times a day in severely painful disorders. Ordinarily, daily injections or interrupted blocks twice a week suffice. In the absence of symptomatic improvement after three treatments, the blocks are discontinued.

Continuous stellate block by means of a polyethylene catheter placed in situ through a hollow needle, carried out for 2 to 3 days in the hospital, is advisable in severe or refractory cases.

SUPRASCAPULAR NERVE BLOCK

Indications

Suprascapular nerve block is rarely employed, because the intrinsic disorders of the shoulder for which it was chiefly used so often respond to local injections of corticosteroids. For suprascapular neuropathy and in subjects not suitable for corticosteroid therapy or X-ray treatment, the method has a place.

Technique

In suprascapular nerve block the patient is placed in the sitting position with the arms hanging at the sides. The hands may rest on the thighs. The head and shoulders are slightly flexed to make the scapula more prominent.

According to the method of Wertheim and Rovenstine, and of Betcher, the superficial landmarks are determined and outlined with a skin-marking pencil. First a line is drawn to mark the upper edge of the base of the spine of the scapula extending from the tip of the acromion to the medial border of the scapular bone (Fig. 5–11, *A-S*). The inferior angle of the scapula is then traced on the skin (*AN*). It is bisected and the bisector is drawn cephalad, crossing the line which marks the base of the spine. The upper outer triangle formed by the intersecting lines is also bisected. On this line a point of 1.5 cm marks the site of introduction of the needle (Wertheim and Rovenstine).

An analgesic wheal is raised, through which a 3-in. 20- or 22-G needle is introduced so that the shaft is directed slightly downward and medially, to make contact with the smooth surface of the supraspinatus fossa lateral

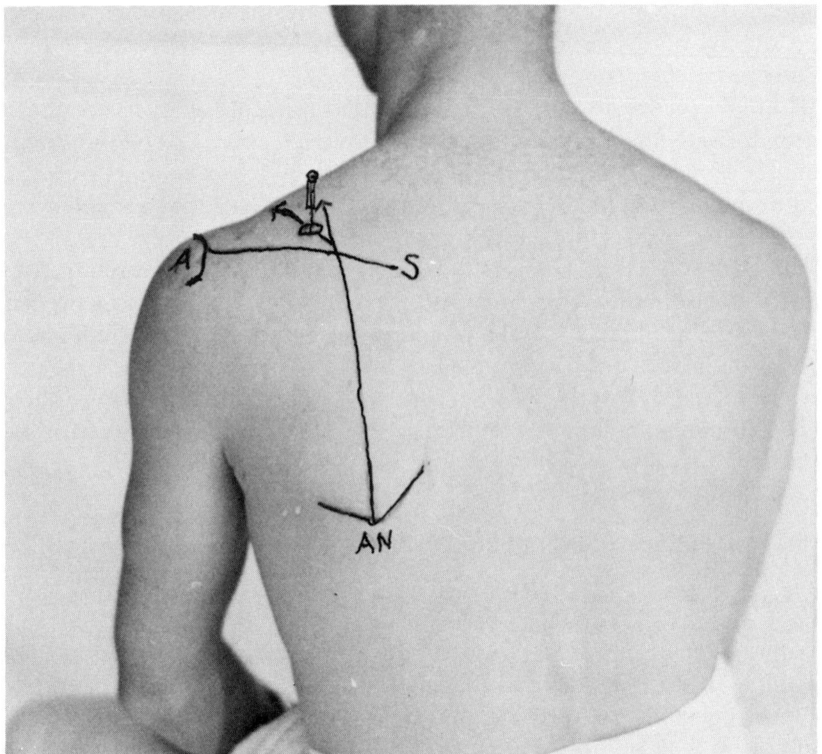

Fig. 5–11. Suprascapular block (after Wertheim and Rovenstine), with its markings. The needle is shown after being reintroduced into the suprascapular notch. *A-S* represents the spine of the scapula from the acromion to the medial border. *A-N* outlines the inferior angle of the scapula. (From Wertheim, HM and Rovenstine, DA. *Anesthesiology* 2: 541, 1941.)

to the notch above the suprascapular fossa. In this position the needle will be in contact with the medial extremity of the base of the coracoid process. The needle shaft is marked with mercurochrome or iodine at a point 1 cm from the skin surface and it is reintroduced medially until the point enters the notch (Fig. 5–10). Radiating paresthesias may accompany contact with the nerve, the maximum intensity of which occurs at the apex of the shoulder. Aspiration is done to be sure the needle is not in a blood vessel.

For therapeutic purposes 5 ml of 1 per cent lidocaine suffices as an initial injection. Relief of pain should follow within 5 to 10 minutes. Thereafter 5 to 10 ml of 1 or 2% lidocaine are given at 3- to 7-day intervals, or longer, depending on the severity of the pain and the patient's response. Graded shoulder exercises are added when pain has diminished.

6

The Upper Limb

THE ARM MUSCLES

A variety of pains arise directly from the anatomical constituents of the arm muscles. Others merely radiate along their neural distribution, running down from the shoulder area, or from the cervical spine.

Pain in the upper or lower part of the arm, usually in the musculature, is our chief concern here. Pain is a common source of complaint. Often, after further questioning or examination, the pain is found to radiate from a lesion at the shoulder area or from pathology at the cervical spine, with further symptoms appearing in the upper part of the extremity, and possibly also in the fingers.

Tender points, which may be of local origin due to circumscribed irritability, are often demonstrable. The local tenderness may be spotty and may represent, or be continuous with, soreness associated with a wider distribution. Not infrequently, diffuse hyperesthesia occurs around the muscles. Systemic conditions also give similar symptoms here.

Local muscular pain, with delimited tenderness, may arise from trauma, strain, or from the various other sources of local soreness. The deltoid, biceps, and other muscles of the arm may be the sites of trigger or tender points.

The shoulder joint and its adjacent structures often are the location of projected symptoms caused by emotional disorders. The arm and shoulder may present diffuse or patchy cutaneous hyperesthesia. The hyperesthesia may be demarcated and represent the distribution of peripheral neuritis or radiculopathy which must be identified.

Local injection of lidocaine alone or with corticosteroid sometimes is carried out in the muscles of each area for nonspecific or posttraumatic lesions of localized character. The shoulder area is a "busy" anatomical crossroads where pain may be referred from the thoracic viscera, the cervical spine, and cerebrospinal disorders. Careful differentiation is often required here.

THE ELBOW REGION

The elbow is subject to frequently occurring, characteristic forms of extraarticular pathology. These consist of a calcific tendinitis at the elbow, or, usually nonspecific medial epicondylitis ("golfers" elbow), lateral epicondylitis ("tennis" elbow), tendinitis at the upper radius or ulna, or combinations of these disorders. The exact cause is unknown, but they often begin at the tendinous insertions at the radius or ulna and the lower end of the humerus producing a tendinitis, and sometimes a radiohumeral bursitis. Trauma is often suspected and undoubtedly is provocative when a latent lesion or symptoms already are present.

Conservative measures may be given a trial. The elbow is soaked for 15 to 20 minutes in hot water with or without epsom salts and then rubbed gently with a liniment or cream for 2 to 3 minutes, daily. Later, gentle exercises are added. If troublesome pain persists, or if improvement is not apparent in a few weeks, local injection is indicated.

In lateral or medial epicondylitis there is usually prolonged pain, with a history of inability to hold a moderately heavy object with the elbow level. This may be confirmed by special tests. The point of maximum tenderness makes the most suitable site for injection. Sometimes a few of these locations are sore and seem to contribute to the discomfort.

INJECTION TECHNIQUE

At the visible and prominent medial or lateral (humeral) epicondyle, subcutaneous injection suffices (20 mg prednisolone) (Fig. 6–1).

At the upper anterior radial border especially, a long line of steady or punctate tenderness may be elicited by palpation. Through a skin wheal at the most sensitive point as the center, the tissue is penetrated and part of the preparation is introduced there. The needle is partly withdrawn and still kept subcutaneous, then redirected upward for 0.5 to 1.0 in., then for the same distance below the initial tender point to make a fanwise distribution (Fig. 6–2). If there is a spot sensitivity, without any other, the medication is deposited subcutaneously over it, usually over the humeral epicondyle, or over the periosteal surface at the radius or ulna as they are touched by the needle.

When there is a long line of tenderness, as sometimes happens over

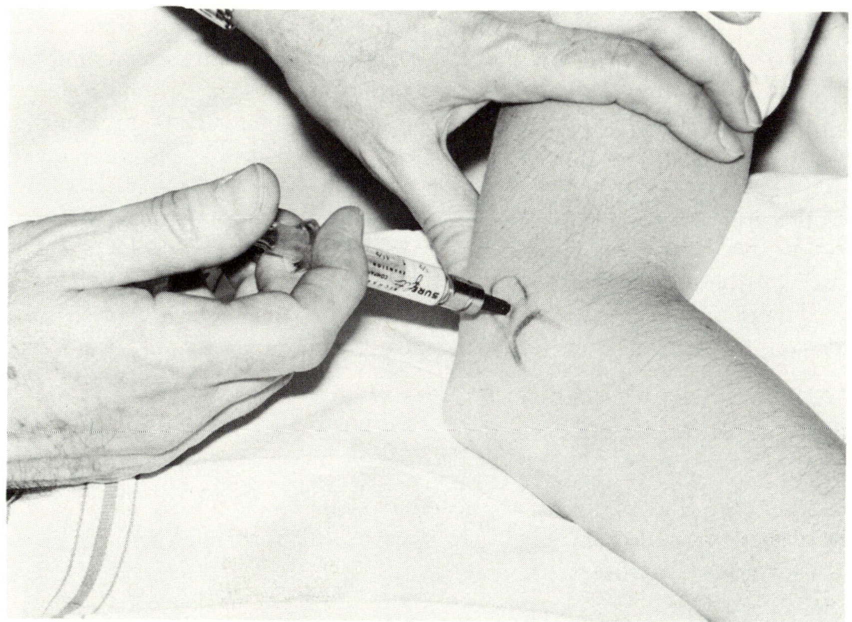

Fig. 6–1. Injection at lateral epicondyle.

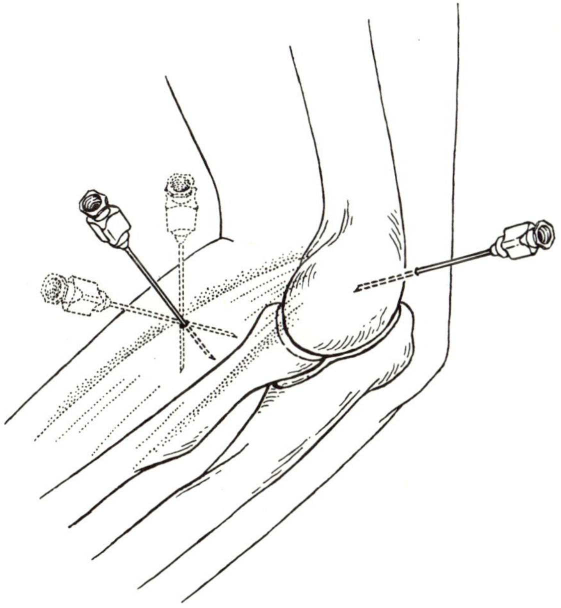

Fig. 6–2. Injection of epicondylitis and variants at the elbow.

the upper end of the radial border, and occasionally over the ulnar, then the fanwise technique is desirable. The dosage depends on the extent of the area to be infiltrated, and ranges from 20 to 50 mg of prednisolone suspension with 2 to 3 ml of lidocaine. One or more injections may be necessary to get lasting results. Sometimes a few sites have to be injected and the total medication divided. It is wise to treat tender points at any of these locations at the same session or in a series of local treatments. Local anesthesia with ethyl chloride spray or with a lidocaine wheal is used for these injections. Mechanical injectors serve well here.

If there is no response within a week, and then longer, after two or three sessions, orthopedic consultation for possible surgery must be considered.

THE ELBOW JOINT

Aspiration and injection of the elbow joint are done usually by the posterolateral approach, where the synovial bulge or tenderness is likely to be found (Fig. 6–3).

INJECTION TECHNIQUE

With the arm incompletely extended and resting, the bulge of the effused synovium is noted posterolaterally, just outside the olecranon

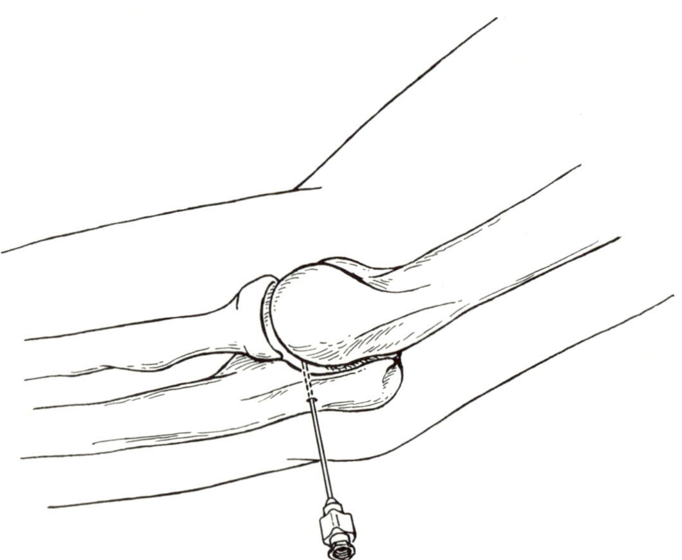

Fig. 6–3. Arthrocentesis of the elbow joint.

process and inferior to the humeral epicondyle. The needle is introduced at the outer side of the olecranon and just below the lateral epicondyle of the humerus. It is directed medially and proximally to the head of the radius. Aspiration, followed by intraarticular injection of 20 to 50 mg of prednisolone suspension, is carried out.

Occasionally, such treatment is necessary for a painful, disabling effusion, chiefly in rheumatoid arthritis, rarely due to trauma.

Olecranon bursitis may resolve spontaneously. When increasingly enlarged and subject to trauma, or tender and inflamed as in rheumatoid disease, provided there is no infection, aspiration and injection with 10 to 25 mg of prednisolone suspension are helpful. If inspissated fluid is expected, a 16- to 18-G needle is necessary for initial aspiration.

Spontaneous, intermittent resolution and recurrence of *subcutaneous nodules* are the rule, with slow asymptomatic enlargement. This benign course does not occur in some cases.

When nodules become tender and larger, especially when exposed to overt trauma and possible infection, they may be responsive to perinodular infiltrations of 10 to 25 mg of prednisolone suspension, according to their size, repeated 1 to 2 times weekly and at longer intervals thereafter, if necessary.

THE WRIST AND ADJACENT TENDONS

Ganglia occur frequently at the hands or feet, especially on the dorsum of the wrist. They consist of cystic swellings containing mucoid material, usually of great density. They may arise along tendon sheaths or about a joint capsule. Spontaneous resolution and recurrence are common. In some cases aspiration and injection of corticosteroid suspension or solution is the treatment of choice. Excision rarely becomes necessary. Recurrence is not infrequent. Our results from aspiration with a large gauge needle (18 G) for thick fluid, followed by introduction of corticosteroid suspension (10 mg) have been generally satisfactory.

The *common dorsal tendon sheath* just distal to the wrist, or other extensor tendon sheaths, may be involved with cystic synovial swelling in rheumatoid arthritis. These fluctuant or boggy prominences may be aspirated, if large enough, followed by instillation of corticosteroid suspension through the same needle, in a dosage of approximately 10 to 25 mg of prednisolone suspension or an equivalent. If fluid is not to be aspirated, a peritendinous injection may be made. Repeated two to six injections at increasing intervals may be required for prolonged control or resolution. Surgery must be considered when recurrences continue to take place, or when increasing periods of relief do not follow after two or

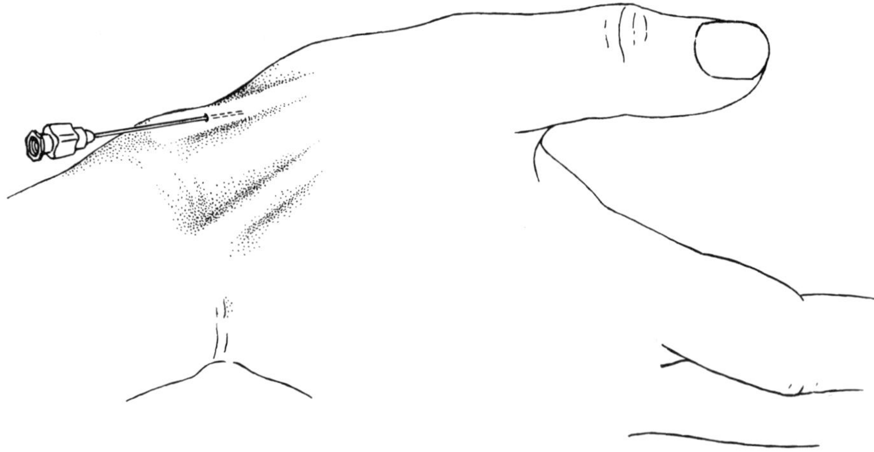

Fig. 6–4. Injection of or at the abductor tendon sheath of the thumb.

three injections, especially in an inflammatory destructive process, such as rheumatoid arthritis.

Tenoysnovitis of the abductor tendon of the thumb (De Quervain's syndrome) is associated with crepitation, sometimes soreness, during motions of the thumb, tenderness to palpation over the abductor tendon inferior to the styloid process of the radius, or over it, and a positive Finkelstein test. The moving tendon usually is visible and palpable under the skin below the styloid process of the radius. There may be swelling. Needling is done at the most tender point, usually below or over the radial styloid process. With or without skin wheals a peritendinous injection with a 0.5-in. 25-G needle is made under the skin with 0.5 ml of lidocaine and 10 to 25 mg of prednisolone suspension (Fig. 6–4).

Only when a visible or palpable sizable effusion occurs into the sheath of the tendon, is the effort made to penetrate the sheath for aspiration and injection.

The injection may be repeated twice a week the first week, then once a week, then at increasing intervals, as the symptoms require, for 2 to 6 sessions. A lightweight splint may be used at night. Long-term effectiveness occurs in 50 to 60% of cases. If there is no improvement, orthopedic consultation should be obtained for possible surgery.

The *median carpal tunnel syndrome* is characterized by pain localized at the wrist, sometimes radiating upward, associated with uncomfortable paresthesias in all or any of the first through the radial half of the fourth fingers but sparing the little finger. Palmar sensory disturbances are found in the distribution of the median nerve. Tenderness to palpation at the base of the thumb may be demonstrated; frequently a positive Tinel's

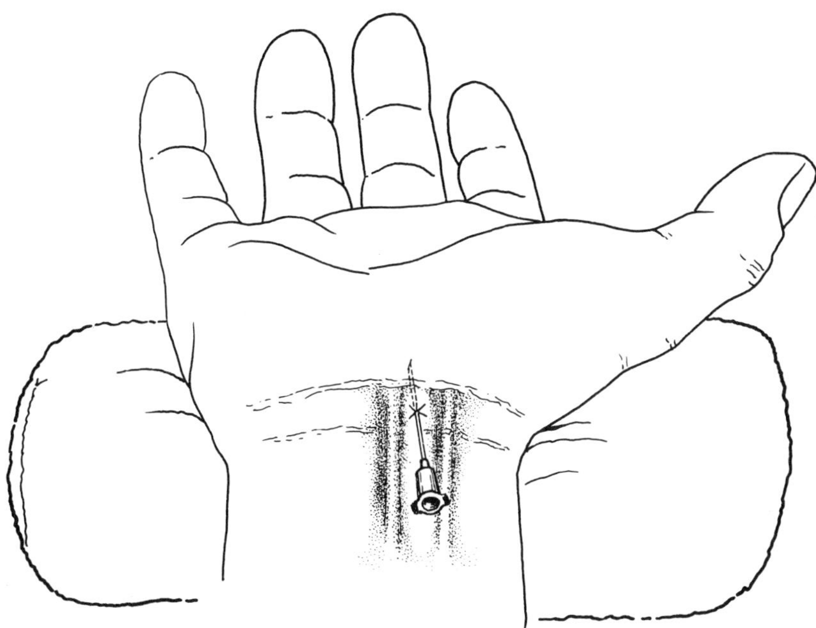

Fig. 6–5. Injection of the median carpal tunnel, the wrist dorsiflexed over a rolled towel.

sign is elicited by tapping over the median nerve at the volar surface of the wrist. Severe atrophy of the thenar eminence may be visible, and with this sign present surgical intervention must be seriously considered.

The carpal tunnel may be injected by inserting the needle with the hand dorsiflexed over a towel or a piece of sponge rubber (Fig. 6–5). A wheal of lidocaine or a freezing point of ethyl chloride spray is raised just medial to the palmaris longus tendon and proximal to the distal transverse crease at the wrist (Fig. 6–5). A 1-in., 22- to 24-G needle is used, directed at an angle of 60° to the skin, pointing distally. The needle is advanced approximately 1 to 2 cm until little or no resistance to the injection is encountered. Prednisolone suspension 25 to 50 mg, with 0.5 ml of lidocaine are injected along the track and into the space. Nocturnal discomfort may be promptly relieved. Paresthesias may require 1 to 2 weeks to abate. Up to four injections may be required at weekly or longer intervals. If symptoms are refractory or recurrent, surgery to decompress the median nerve is indicated.

Aspiration and injection of the wrist joint are through the bulging synovial membrane when it is distended (Hollander, 1966; Miller, 1956; Findler and Post; Neustadt, 1963). Tender, soft tissues at articular sites are usually suitable points of entry. There may be one or several such loca-

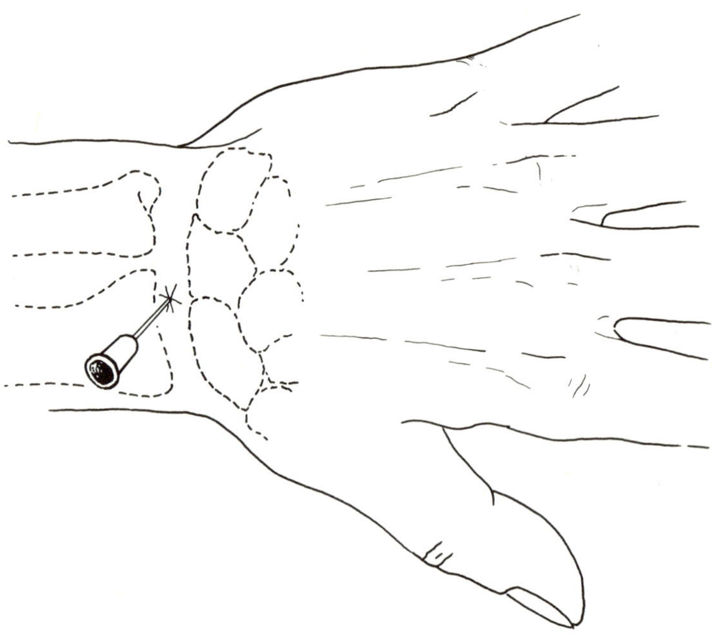

Fig. 6–6. Arthrocentesis of the wrist, radial or lateral entry.

tions characteristic of inflammation of this joint. The chief points of entry are radial and ulnar, generally prominent on account of effusion or swelling.

Radial or lateral entry is made at the dorsum of the wrist with the hand somewhat flexed over a rolled towel, most commonly at a point on the dorsum just medial to the extensor tendon of the thumb just below the distal border of the radius at its midpoint (Fig. 6–6).

The ulnar or medial entry of the joint space may be made by inserting the needle into the space just below the lateral ulnar margin in the palpable gap between this border and the carpus (Fig. 6–7). Aspiration is carried out at any or each of these points through a skin wheal or frozen point with a 0.5 to 1 in., 22- 20-G needle; 10 to 25 mg of prednisolone suspension with or without 0.5 ml of lidocaine solution instilled at either or both portions of the joint.

Inflammation at adjacent intercarpal spaces and carpometacarpal joints, especially at the first, or between the carpus and the other parts of the wrist, are reflected by tender points and sites of bulging at or near the wrist. If troublesome, the affected locus usually is more tender, possibly fluctuant. It can be entered at its prominence or most tender point, aspirated if possible, then 5 to 25 mg of prednisolone are introduced into (if the needle tip slides in readily) or about it.

Surface anesthesia at the wrist and finger joints is provided by ethyl

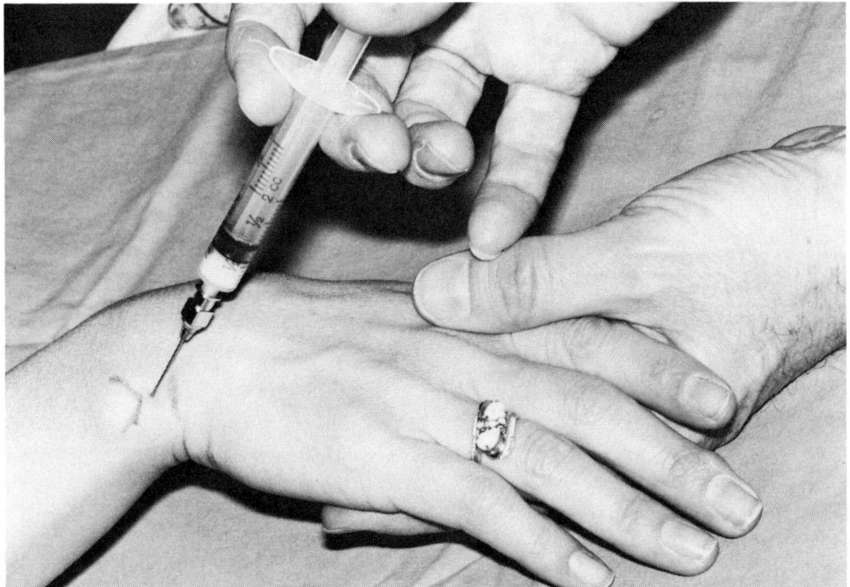

Fig. 6–7. Arthrocentesis and injection of the wrist, ulnar entry.

chloride spray to produce a freezing point of entry. The skin is sensitive or thin at the palm and at the sides of finger joints especially, for skin wheals with a needle. Mechanical injectors are notably useful for these joints.

The freezing wheal or point of entry is placed slightly away from the usually exquisitely tender point. After the needle tip gets under the skin it is directed to the actual point of tenderness or swelling or teased into the articular space.

TENOSYNOVITIS OF DIGITAL FLEXOR TENDONS

In tenosynovitis of digital flexor tendons ("trigger" or "snapping" finger), the usual catch of the tendon in its sheath is due to inflammation, swelling of the tendon and/or a fibrinous deposit at a point in the tendon sheath, at the base of a metacarpophalangeal joint, the usual site where the snapping occurs. The condition may be mild or severe. The patient may have to complete flexion or extension of the finger with the other hand. Tenderness to palpation at the distal head of the corresponding metacarpal in the line of the flexor tendon overlying it is a characteristic clinical feature; this is the site for local injection.

Spontaneous recovery is not rare if the patient is willing to wait and

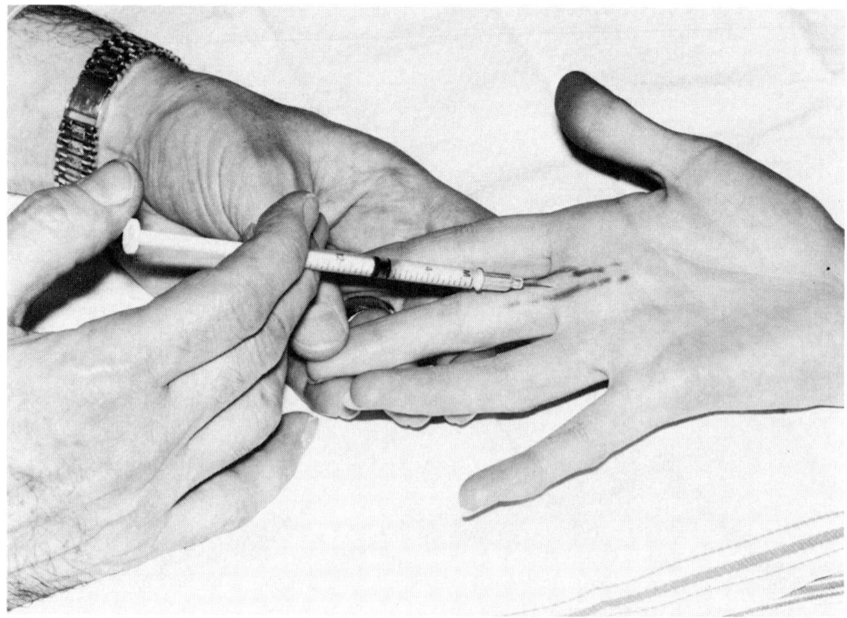

Fig. 6–8. Injection of or at the flexor tendon sheath of the third finger.

finds no interference with work. It is possible that other flexor tendons may be affected later. The authors have seen four of five flexor tendons involved successively.

In mild conditions of recent onset, local soaks in warm epsom salt solution for 15 to 20 minutes, twice a day, a night splint to keep the finger straight, and sponge-squeezing exercises may be tried for 4 to 8 weeks. If there is no response to this regimen local injection is warranted. For longstanding, unresponsive cases, infiltration therapy is initiated at once.

The point of maximum tenderness at the distal head of the corresponding metacarpal of the affected flexor tendon is infiltrated without anesthesia or through a point frozen with ethyl chloride spray, penetrated with a 0.5-in. 25-G needle for an injection of 0.25 ml (12.5 mg) of prednisolone suspension, or its equivalent, which may be mixed with 0.25 ml of lidocaine (Fig. 6–8). This is given subcutaneously, or peritendinally by injecting the medication just to one side of the sheath of the flexor tendon, if possible. Repeat injections from 2 to 6 days or at intervals of 5 to 10 days or more are usually effective and lasting in 50 to 60% of the cases.

When a contraindicatioin to corticosteroids exists, injection of lidocaine alone is often effective, but requires a longer program of treatment to be beneficial.

Surgery is indicated for refractory cases.

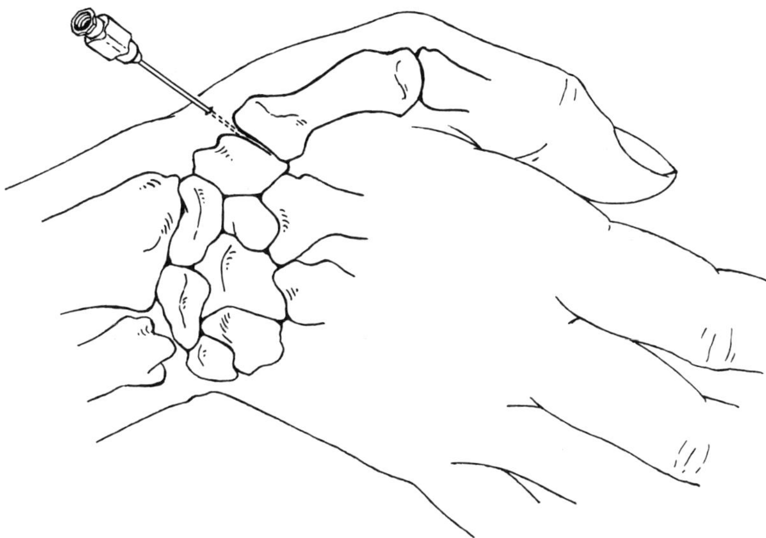

Fig. 6–9. Arthrocentesis of the carpometacarpal joint of the thumb.

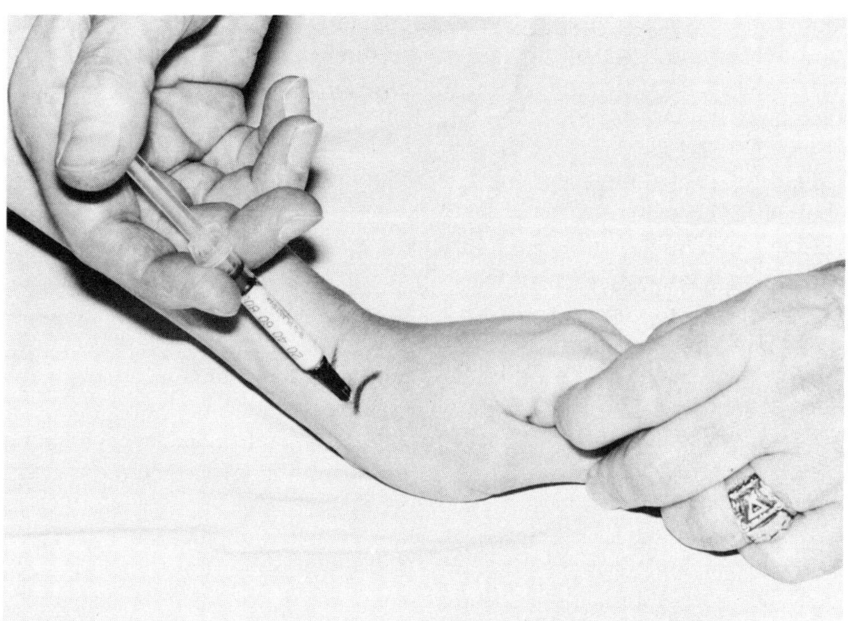

Fig. 6–10. Actual entry of the carpometarcarpal joint of the thumb.

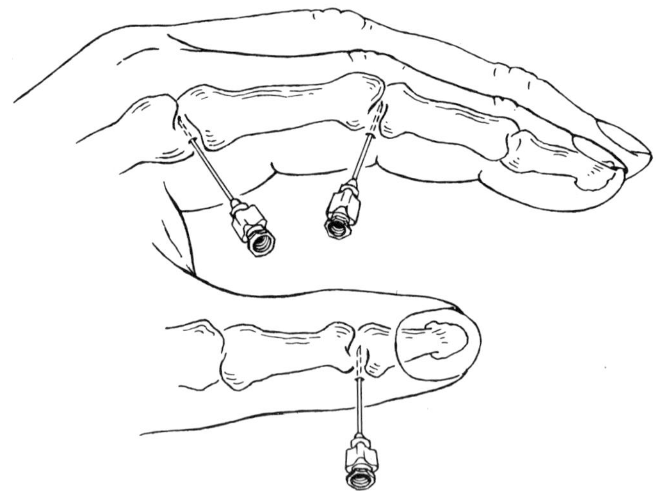

Fig. 6–11. Arthrocentesis of the joints of the fingers.

THE FINGER JOINTS

The carpometacarpal joints sometimes require injection, and the method follows that used for the proximal interphalangeals. The carpometacarpal joint of the thumb is that most often affected (thumb base osteoarthritis). It is entered dorsally from the radial side of the thumb at the point of maximum tenderness, with the thumb held in flexion within the palm (Figs. 6–9 and 6–10).

The proximal interphalangeal (PIP) joints are frequently involved in rheumatoid arthritis. In these small joints it is necessary to use a gentle teasing technique to enter the joint (Figs. 6–11 and 6–12). When the joint is swollen, with distention of the capsule, it suffices to approach the articulation laterally or medially with a 25- to 27-G needle, with or without a wheal just below the dorsal surface. Rather than attempt to get into the tiny joint space, the needle is insinuated gently into the bulging capsule. When there is no true bulging, simple pericapsular and subcutaneous injection without painful attempts to enter the joint have, in our experience, sufficed. Apparently, ready transport of the corticosteroid occurs through inflamed capsule and synovia.

When aspiration is attempted, it requires a fine needle, such as 23 to 26 G, and a 2-ml syringe. Vigorous efforts to aspirate fluid are not justified except to obtain a few drops for culture, if infection is suspected. Whether or not effusion is aspirated, the injection of medication is completed. A mixture of 0.25 ml of lidocaine with 12.5 mg of prednisolone

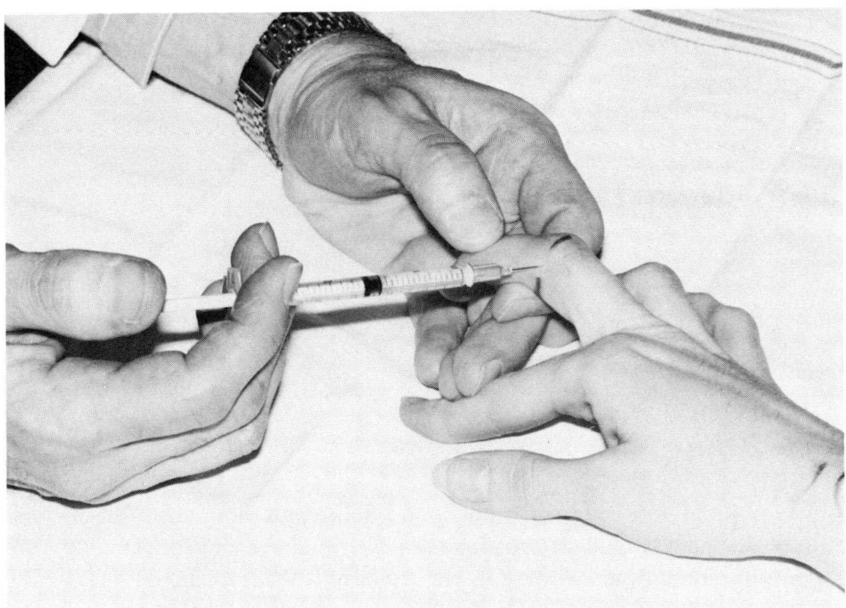

Fig. 6–12. Injection of a proximal interphalangeal joint.

suspension (0.25 ml) is instilled. When several joints are involved, two or three procedures may be done at one session provided the patient can tolerate them. In these approaches we infiltrate small, tight, structures with a capacity for only a small amount of fluid.

The distal interphalangeal joints may be affected by inflammatory synovitis, as in psoriasis, synovitis of degenerative joint disease, or by a reactive, local inflammation superimposed on a degenerative joint process (Heberden's nodes). Mucous cysts associated with Heberden's nodes at the dorsum of the affected joint can be "unroofed," inspissated fluid aspirated, and a small dose of corticosteroid suspension instilled.

Aspiration and injection at the distal joints are carried out by the method used for the proximal joints.

The Dermo-Jet and Hypospray devices are useful for injections at the tendons and joints of the fingers and for the intercarpal spaces.

7

The Chest Regions

The role of intrathoracic and spondylotic pathology should be considered in analyzing the origin of pain in the chest wall or its radiation. Upper abdominal pathology must be excluded. With localized chest pain, lesions of the ribs must be borne in mind, particularly in middle-aged or elderly people, notably those with skeletal demineralization. Past or recent fracture, without overt trauma, is not an unusual source of local discomfort. Exquisite tenderness, sharply localized, is significant. If there is definite increase of pain on mobility of the chest frame without a demonstrable basis, it should be an indication for radiography. Usually, before undertaking any injection therapy in the chest area, it is wise to have chest X-ray films, and occasionally spinal films, as well as deliberate evaluation of the complaints. A patient with suspicious chest pain should have an electrocardiogram.

THE ANTERIOR CHEST

Circumscribed points tender to palpation may be located in the chest wall in muscles, and fibrolipomatous and other subcutaneous structures. In apprehensive individuals, particularly those subject to angina, diffuse cutaneous hyperesthesia may be demonstrable, requiring evaluation of its role in response to local injection therapy.

Costochondritis (Tietze's syndrome) is a nonspecific inflammatory process, usually of the upper sternocostal cartilages, especially the second, which may become persistently painful. The condition is usually self-limiting and is managed with simple measures. In unresponsive cases, local subcutaneous injections with a 0.5- to 1.0-in., 25-G needle at each point of tenderness of 1 to 2 ml of Xylocaine with 10 to 20 mg of cortico-

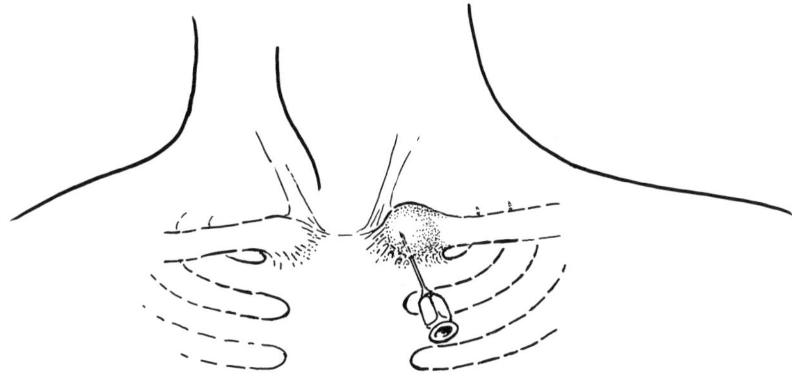

Fig. 7–1. Arthrocentesis of the sternoclavicular joint.

steroid suspension may prove effective. Repeated infiltration may be necessary.

Acromioclavicular arthropathy is symptomatic chiefly from soft tissue irritation or swelling at this joint. If unresponsive to simple measures, it may be benefited by injection. The joint is located by palpation. Through a wheal a 22-G needle is inserted at the tender point or margins and directed straight down between the latter until it is felt to slide (*see* Fig. 5–2*C*). A dose of 10 to 20 mg of prednisolone suspension with or without 0.5 ml of lidocaine is used.

Sternoclavicular arthropathy may be degenerative or inflammatory. Arthritic involvement may produce painful enlargement. If no contraindication is found, the often visible or palpable capsulitis, when not responsive to other measures, may be aspirated and injected with lidocaine (0.5 to 1.0 ml) and 10 to 25 mg of prednisolone suspension. The point of entry is the soft, visible, or palpable bulge overlying the joint subcutaneously (Fig. 7–1).

THE POSTERIOR CHEST

At the posterior thoracic area palpable, tender points, myalgic spots, or circumscribed soreness of the musculature and soft tissues are sometimes found. Paravertebral and parascapular tender points, as well as tender spots in the supraspinatus and infraspinatus area at the scapula are demonstrable by palpation in some cases. When these are circumscribed and show a reliable reaction to palpation without overlying, diffuse cutaneous hyperesthesia, local injection may be effective.

The scapulocostal syndrome of Michele is characterized chiefly by a tender point just under the medial angle of the scapula or adjacent to the medial scapular border that is usually found when the hand of the affected side is brought to the opposite shoulder (Michele *et al.*) We have observed such a localization of tenderness at times; in some patients good results may be obtained by injecting this tender point (in addition to other corrective, postural measures already prescribed).

A test injection of 5 ml of 0.5% lidocaine, subcutaneously at any tender spot, yielding relief, may be followed by 5 to 10 ml of 1% lidocaine alone or with 3 to 5 ml mixed with 10 to 20 mg prednisolone suspension, depending on how sharply defined is the tenderness. Various localizations of tender points are encountered in poor posture, overweight, overburdened, and disturbed subjects. Control saline infiltration tests are useful.

The above holds true also for the various myalgic spots found along the spinal muscles under similar circumstances. It is quite possible that often enough such points of tenderness arise from past trauma, continuing occupational stresses, the mechanical strain of poor posture and unnatural positions during work or at rest which put a steady load on these areas, often in patients with spinal alterations. In some cases an element of nervous tension may be associated with the complaints.

LOCAL INJECTION THERAPY

Local injection can be carried out at any of the circumscribed tender sites, frequently with good results and often without the addition of corticosteroids. Local injection of 2 to 5 ml of 0.5% lidocaine, later 1%, may give relief and may require repetition a few times. If an inflammatory lesion is suspected, 10 or 20 mg of prednisolone suspension may be mixed with the lidocaine. Occasionally, such localized sites of inflammation or irritation may occur in patients with systemic disease, such as rheumatoid arthritis, ankylosing spondylitis, or osteoarthritis, as well as in disorders with no demonstrable cause.

Observation of the effect of an intracutaneous wheal and of subcutaneous normal saline as a first or second injection may prove useful as a control for evaluation of the patient's response, suggestibility, or placebo reactor state.

INTERCOSTAL NEURALGIA

Pain in a costal or intercostal distribution from the posterior thoracic to the lateral and anterior chest, or in segmental patterns, is consistent with an intercosal neuralgia.

Intercostal nerve block is indicated if standard analgesic measures have failed, provided no underlying pathology is responsible.

SEGMENTAL NEURALGIAS OR NEUROPATHIES

Various segmental neuralgias and neuropathies arising anywhere along the whole length of the spine may be due to involvement of intraspinal, paraspinal, or radicular elements, or of the nerve trunks prior to branching into their divisions. Such pain may be due to reactive changes of soft tissues lying near the intervertebral foramina and their proximate nerve trunks.

Neuralgias of the cervical, thoracic, and lumbosacral areas are not uncommon, and arise from irritative, discogenic, or hypertrophic changes about or at the nerve roots. They may be caused by inflammatory reactions of the soft tissues surrounding one or more of the nerve roots or nerves coursing along the intercostal spaces or transmitted via the affected radicular structures. The latter may be associated with or follow upper respiratory infections, muscular strain, and rheumatoid or other systemic musculoskeletal conditions. In these segmental disorders there may be a definite distribution along the dermatomes of the skin, sometimes with other neurologic signs, giving the localization, origin, and distribution of pain corresponding to the segmental neural involvement. X-ray films may assist in, or confirm, localization. Occasionally, a neoplasm is responsible.

Management

Conservative measures of the basic program are directed to the pain and the underlying cause. If these fail, nerve blocks and orthopedic aids or supports may be indicated (Bonica, 1964).

Post-herpetic neuralgia occasionally presents refractory painful symptoms. Paravertebral sympathetic nerve blocks may be used. The symptoms may respond to repeated infiltration subcutaneously of lidocaine 1% up to 20 ml in large areas, under the peripheral distribution of the eruption and the tender, painful area. The addition of 2 mg of triamcinolone in suspension per ml, with reasonable total quantities, has been found to give prolonged effects when infiltrated subcutaneously under the peripheral lesions (Epstein).

8

Low Back Pain

Low back pain is a common form of musculoskeletal discomfort. This area includes the musculoskeletal structures of the back from the lowest dorsal vertebra to the coccyx. The pain may be localized, or it may be associated with sciatic radiation or other radicular symptoms and distribution.

Low back pain may be of varying severity and duration, and range from acute to subacute to chronic intensity. Naturally, many conditions of the supportive structures in this area produce the variable "symptoms of soft tissue lesions," from postural strain to disorders of discs, vertebrae, and intervertebral joints. Other pathology may provoke the intervertebral soft tissues or the perispinal muscular structures, including the nerve roots. These give the clinical picture of soft tissue lesions, especially nerve root irritation.

Troublesome discomfort may arise from a number of causes and may originate in any of the structures of the lumbosacral area. Obviously, to attack the superficial features of some underlying disease, such as spondylitis or extensive osteoarthritis of the spine, without a correct working diagnosis and an appropriate therapeutic program, is not apt to be rewarding.

INJECTION TREATMENT

Before undertaking injection therapy for low back symptoms, it is wise to review the various causes.

In the differentiation and evaluation of symptoms it must be borne in mind that pain in the low back and in the lower extremities may be produced by cervical spinal cord compression in rare cases. The role of spondylosis, spondylarthrosis, and discogenic irritation or compression of nerve roots in the lumbar spine in painful disorders of the low back and extremities should be considered. Neurologic or orthopedic consultation may be necessary in some cases.

Techniques for the treatment of low back pain include the following: ethyl chloride (or other vapocoolant) spray; local injection of soft tissue lesions; injection of gluteal-parasciatic tender points; peritrochanteric injection; paravertebral blocks of spinal nerves or sympathetic ganglia; caudal block; coccygeal injections; bursal injection; and injection of painful fat pads. All of these will be discussed in turn below.

Skin wheals and saline injections are used effectively in the low back region, as controls and to evaluate responses.

LOCALIZATIONS

Various localizations of these soft tissue disturbances or reflected pathology may be found in the low back, as discussed above for the neck and shoulder area (see Chapters 4 and 5). Low back disturbances may arise de novo or serve as symptoms of some underlying localized or systemic musculoskeletal pathology, with neural and/or muscular components. Tender points and trigger points may be found at any of the accessible muscles or other structures of the supportive tissues. The relationship of these symptoms to coexisting vertebral pathology must be carefully distinguished.

SUBCUTANEOUS AND DEEPER SOFT TISSUE DISORDERS

Superficial or deep soreness to palpation may be found in the area of the paravertebral, gluteal, and other lumbosacral muscles, and supportive structures.

A coexisting, often secondary, soft tissue lesion or irritative reaction in spondylosis or other spinal disorder may be caused by persistent postural deficiency, strain, or other disturbed functions of the tissues of the low back. Occasionally, the symptomatology is the result of long-standing, localized, or superficial, irritative and feedback reactions. It is effective in some of these conditions to inject the tender, accessible myofascial manifestations. Suppression or relief of symptoms may be expedited, especially when the basic deficiency or disease is corrected or treated at the same time.

Ethyl Chloride Spray

Ethyl chloride spray may be beneficial to patients who are subject to moderate low back pain and muscular spasm (especially when acute).

A safe technique is to make ten to fifteen 5- to 6-in. passes over the painful or sore area, without frosting. These may be repeated. A gentle massage with an analgesic balm or liniment may reinforce the response.

ACUTE LOW BACK PAIN

Acute low back pain may be discogenic or radicular, traumatic or commonly idiopathic, so-called acute lumbago, characterized by diffuse soft tissue soreness.

LOW BACK PAIN WITH OR WITHOUT SCIATICA

Low back pain with or without sciatica is a common disorder seen by the clinician. Neoplasm, disc syndrome, radiculopathies, spinal arthropathies, chronic postural strain and all of the etiologies, major and minor, must be considered in the evaluation of the symptoms.

Low back pain without any evidence of underlying disease, with or without sciatic radiation, unresponsive to conservative measures (e.g., analgesics, a bed board or other support, local heat, rest, and traction) may be relieved by local injections if there are tender points to palpation. The soreness to palpation may be diffuse in one or a few areas. If there is no tenderness to palpation, local injection is not likely to be beneficial.

Local Injection of Soft Tissue Lesions

Local injection of the most tender points with 10 ml of 0.5% lidocaine (divided among two to three spots if equally tender) is often effective. The injection may be repeated with 1 per cent solution at intervals of 2 to 3 days or longer for three sessions. It should supplement the conservative measures mentioned above. When there is a definite benefit, repeated injection is warranted should pain recur. If there are no contraindications and response to the local anesthetic is inadequate or of short duration, 25 to 30 mg of prednisolone suspension, or its equivalent, may be added to the analgesic solution for infiltration of the tender points. The more circumscribed the points of tenderness, the less the amount of lidocaine needed (2 to 5 ml as a rule) at any sharply demarcated point.

SCIATICA OR SCIATICA-LIKE SYNDROME

Sciatica or the sciatica-like syndrome consists chiefly of low back pain, tenderness of the muscles of the area, or in tenderness in the region of the sciatic notch with slight or marked radiation along the distribution of the sciatic nerve. Tenderness often is demonstrable by palpation medially at the gluteal area, or in the upper or lower portion of the gluteal region. Any added positive neurologic signs have important diagnostic significance, whether reflex, sensory, or motor. Motor weakness or impaired reflexia requires careful consideration of the underlying cause.

Gluteal-Parasciatic Injection

Local injection of the most tender point is indicated. As already mentioned, repeated injections may be necessary at a depth sufficient to infiltrate the tender tissues. It is desirable to proceed cautiously in advancing the needle deeply into tender points over or close to the sciatic notch, using a needle no longer than 2 inches. The sciatic nerve may be entered at a depth of 2.5 in. or more along the midline of the gluteal and posterior thigh areas over and below the sciatic notch. Patients describe a lightning-like or "electric" pain which radiates down the posterior midline of the limb to the foot.

When this pain occurs, it is necessary to aspirate and withdraw the needle at least 1 to 2 cm from the reactive point before injecting. Otherwise, the sciatic nerve may be anesthetized when its sheath is entered, or if the solution is deposited contiguously. When the solution is adjacent to or within the sheath, it causes a weakness of the extremity of varying intensity lasting 15 to 30 minutes or more, or for the duration of the anesthesia. Since the limb may give way during weight-bearing, the patient must sit or lie down until the anesthesia wears off.

Sciatic nerve injection of any degree is rarely carried out as a therapeutic measure. The transient weakness of the limb that follows such a procedure is disconcerting to the patient, no matter how much assurance is given him in advance. In special cases, it is possible to induce the pain as a signal to determine the point from which to withdraw the needle so as to provide an analgesic effect with little or no motor weakness.

Peritrochanteric Injection

Localizing tender points for injection about the greater trochanter of the femur, described by Breneman, is an effective method in some cases of low back pain and sciatica (Figs. 8–1*A* and *B*). These localized points are found frequently in the disc syndromes and the distal painful disorders of the spinal or perispondylar structures. Injection may be helpful and offers an uncomplicated approach. Breneman has noted palpably tender and indurated points which, when infiltrated, relieve the symptoms. The maximum tender point or trigger point is located by palpation. Two or 3 ml of lidocaine are infiltrated with a 1.5-in., 22-G needle. When the tenderness is abolished, 20 to 40 mg of prednisolone suspension, or its equivalent, is introduced. The procedure may have to be carried out at a few tender points in divided corticosteroid dosage with more lidocaine, and one or more additional treatments may be required.

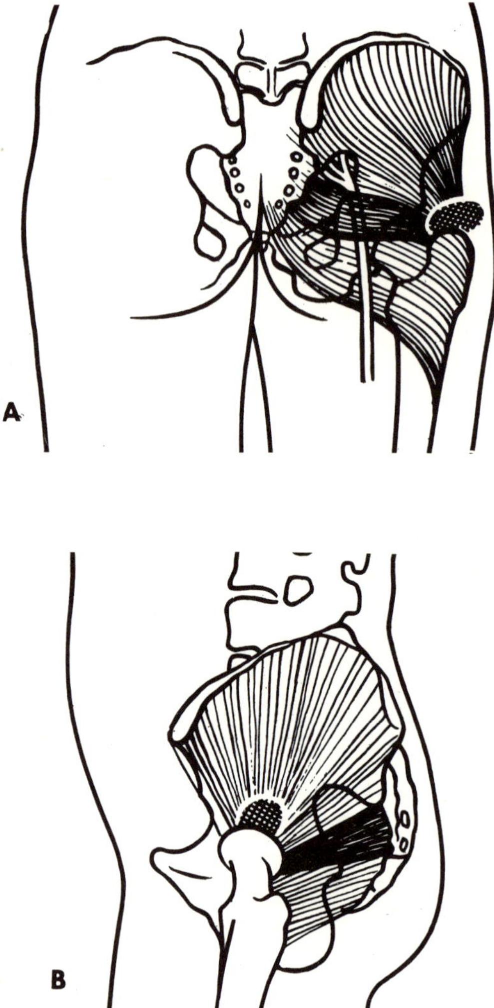

Fig. 8–1. *A*. Peritrochanteric injection site for low back pain. Hatched area is the tender entry site, posterior view. (From Breneman, JC. *J Occup Med 11*: 475, 1969). *B*. Lateral view.

Paravertebral Spinal Nerve Block

Lumbar neuralgia with segmental distribution of cutaneous sensory signs may occur with refractory pain in that region. It may be associated with changes in the tendon reflexes and motor function of the affected muscles.

A variety of spinal pathology, spondylosis or arthritis, juxtaarticular inflammation with nerve root involvement, discogenic disorders, infection, neoplasm, trauma, postural strain, and muscular pathology must be considered among the causes.

Management. When a definite localization with segmental cutaneous distribution occurs, a conservative program should be initiated. If the symptoms are acute and no infectious or malignant cause is identified, such measures may suffice. Bed rest and traction may be required. For pain that persists, nerve block with lidocaine may be helpful. Blocks may be repeated at increasing intervals determined by the patient's responsiveness. In due time, if these various measures fail to provide adequate relief, or if abnormal reflex sensory or motor responses are present, neurologic, neurosurgical, or orthopedic consultation is advisable.

Paravertebral Sympathetic Ganglion Block

Paravertebral lumbar sympathetic ganglion block is indicated in herpetic and postherpetic neuralgia of lumbar segmental distribution, especially in early reflex dystrophy. The procedure has been used for diagnostic, prognostic, and therapeutic evaluation in Raynaud's syndrome, for troublesome pain of the feet or lower extremities unresponsive to the usual measures, and in circulatory disorders, arterial embolism, thrombosis, thrombophlebitis, arterial injuries, and aneurysm.

Caudal Block

Caudal (epidural) block is applied in sciatica and low back pain unresponsive to simple methods, and also in disc syndromes not ready, or suitable, for surgery.

Anatomy. In caudal block the needle is passed through the sacral hiatus and the anesthetic solution is deposited within the sacral canal (outside the dura). The essentials of Labat's method are followed here. The sacral hiatus is an opening resulting from the defective fusion or nonclosure, of the laminae of the last sacral vertebrae, and is covered by a thin layer of fibrous tissue called the sacrococcygeal membrane (*see* Fig. 8–2). The latter is stretched between the sacrum and the coccyx.

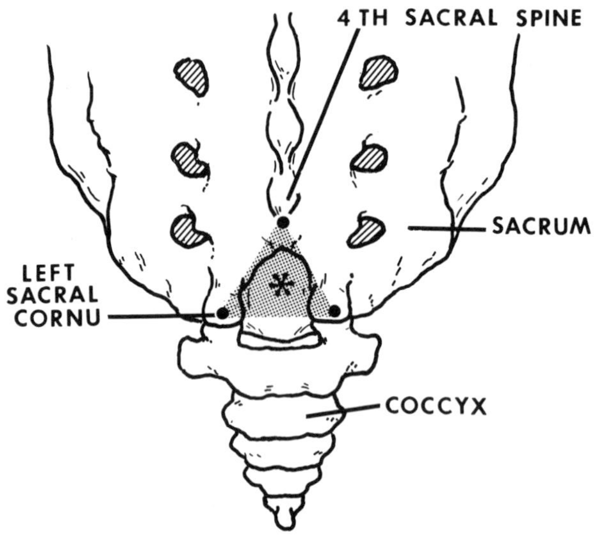

Fig. 8–2. *Epidural injection.* Asterisk marks the site of puncture through the sacral hiatus in the center of the triangle formed by joining the palpable sacral cornua and the fourth sacral spinous process. (After Labat.)

The sacral hiatus lies at the junction of the sacrum and coccyx. It is bounded by the sacral cornua on either side of the spinous process of the fourth sacral vertebra on the midline slightly superior. It has the shape of an inverted V. "The arms of the inverted V are generally salient edges" and their extremities are prominent tubercles, but in some cases these anatomic features cannot be distinguished by palpation. Anomalies of the sacrococcygeal structures occasionally may make caudal block impractical or impossible.

"The sacral canal is filled with loose adipose tissue, richly vascularized," and communicates freely with the epidural space of the lumbar region. The dural sac which lies in the canal contains the lower portion of the cauda equina and in the adult extends as far as the lower border of the second sacral vertebra. The sacral nerves and the coccygeal nerve emerge from the lateral border of the dural sac, close to one another longitudinally, and spread out fanwise to their respective foramina wrapped in individual sheaths extending from the dura.

Technique. The patient lies prone with a cushion placed under his hips to elevate the sacral region. The sacral hiatus is defined by palpating with the tip of the left forefinger from the tip of the coccyx to the sacrococcygeal junction. There the margins are bounded by the sacral

A 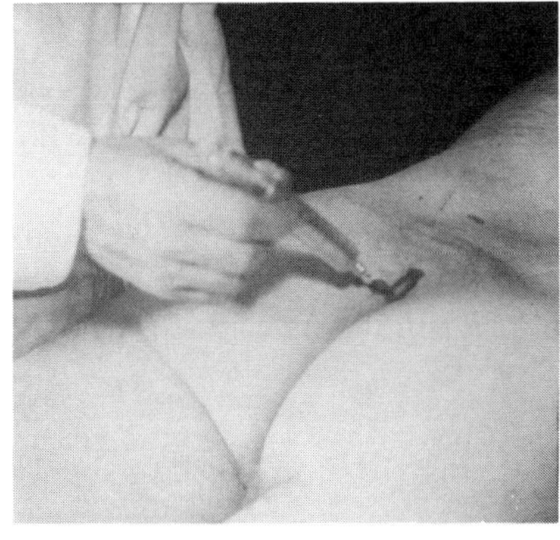

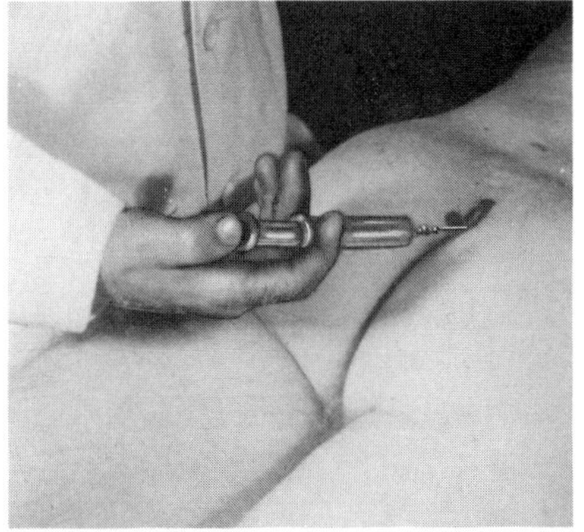 B

Fig. 8–3. *A*. Position of the hand when piercing the sacrococcygeal membrane to enter the caudal canal. *B*. Position of the hand after changing needle direction following entry into the caudal canal.

cornua felt on each side and the fourth sacral spinous process in the midline a little craniad. These three prominences form the angles of a triangular surface through the midpoint of which the needle is introduced with ease (Fig. 8–2).

A fine, spinal puncture needle is used with stylet intact and its bevel turned upward against the posterior wall of the canal. The needle is introduced at a 20° angle through a wheal raised at this point. After penetrating the sacrococcygeal membrane (which, stretching across the sacral hiatus, closes the lower end of the sacral canal) the point of the needle strikes the anterior wall of the canal (Fig. 8–3*A*). It is then withdrawn 1 or 2 cm and the hub of the needle is swung downward toward the gluteal cleft until it is almost level with the body surface (Fig. 8–3*B*).The needle then is advanced in the midline 2 to 4 cm.

Aspiration is carried out and time is allowed to make sure that no blood or spinal fluid returns. In such cases the needle is drawn back a few cm until the flow ceases and the syringe, filled with solution, is connected with the needle. This test is made before injecting the fluid, and makes certain that no intraspinal or intravenous injection is done. The solution is then injected very slowly, using a total of 15 to 20 ml, of 1 per cent lidocaine solution followed by normal saline in increments of 10 ml. As in any of these injection procedures it is advisable to start with 5 cc of 0.5 per cent at first, followed 10 to 15 minutes later by another 5 ml of 0.5%. This tests for tolerance. Thereafter the most desirable quantity for effectiveness may be used (Brown).

The solution should flow freely and without great pressure. The fingers of the free hand rest over the sacrum to detect any tumefaction. If swelling occurs over the dorsal surafce of the sacrum, it indicates that the needle is outside the canal. It should be withdrawn and reinserted.

Unsatisfactory results and failures may be due to the following, according to Labat, as enumerated by him:

1. Inability to enter the sacral canal through lack of knowledge of the anatomic variations of the sacrococcygeal region.
2. Impossibility of entering the canal through absence of accurate landmarks.
3. Decreased permeability of the neural sheath through the sacrum and other nerves.
4. Injection of too weak solutions.
5. Increased capacity of the sacral canal, due to the size of the bone.
6. Defective position of the needle in the canal.
7. Bleeding within the canal, as a result of accidental trauma inflicted by the needle during its penetration.
8. Defective closure of the sacral canal, rendering its penetration and injection dangerous.
9. Injection in the posterior aspect of the sacrum.
10. Impermeability of the sacral hiatus.

COCCYGODYNIA

Coccygodynia may be caused by injury to the sacrococcygeal articulation, or to the surrounding abundant connective tissue of the sacrococcygeal structures. In some cases a rectal examination will reveal a movable coccyx. Former immobility enhances the likelihood of injury. X-ray films may be informative, especially for trauma or infection.

It is not unusual to encounter pain referred to the coccyx, or tenderness over it, whether or not it is movable at the joint. The role of the patient's emotional state in coccygeal complaints must be considered in evaluation and management.

A conservative program, including a coccygeal cushion, should be tried for a reasonable period. If neurotic features are prominent, or if refractoriness raises the question of a psychalgia, neuropsychiatric screening is advisable. If pain and tenderness continue with no demonstrable infection, injury, or associated pathology, subcutaneous and periarticular injections given at the tender point of the area are worth a trial.

Coccygeal Injection

The soreness of the coccyx and the response of the symptoms to local injection at the tender area may be evaluated first with a lidocaine wheal, followed by normal saline injected subcutaneously. If ineffective, these are followed by fanwise injection of 5 ml of 1% lidocaine, rarely later with 10 to 20 mg of prednisolone suspension or its equivalent. Cleanliness and asepsis here are important, especially when corticosteroid suspensions are used. (A sterile cotton ball is placed between the gluteal surfaces to catch any fluid dripping toward the anus.)

Bursal Injections

Bursae of the low back are in most cases located over bony prominences. Sometimes they may be inflamed, painful, and occasionally filled with inspissated material. It is not unusual to find an indurated, cyst-like thickening or nodule over the posterior superior ischial spine, asymptomatic and nontender. These structures at times become enlarged, inflamed, and painful. Subcutaneous nodules may be found adjacent to these locations in patients with rheumatoid arthritis. When cysts, bursae, or nodules are discovered incidentally, are asymptomatic and not tender to palpation, they should be noted, but no action is indicated. When they are painful, swollen, tender, and especially if they contain fluid, they are readily aspirated and injected with 1 to 3 ml of lidocaine, and/or 10 to 20 mg of prednisolone or its equivalent. An attempt should be made to aspirate any fluid before injecting through the intact needle. Perilesional infiltration is carried out when fluid is not obtained.

Ischial bursae may be found at the ischial tuberosities. The trauma of prolonged sitting, especially in lean subjects, direct injury, and inflammation, as in rheumatoid arthritis or degenerative changes are most often responsible (Françon). Here too, when pain and tenderness are found, similar aspiration and injection, perilesional or intralesional, are carried out.

It is important in these areas to be sure no break in the overlying skin indicative of possible infection has occurred.

Injection of Painful Fat Pads

Herniated fat lobules, erupting through their capsules and through the overlying fascia, usually in the low back, have been described as sources of some "fibrositic" pain (Copeman). Local injection rarely is effective. Such recurrent and troublesome lobules, when convincingly demonstrated, have been reportedly excised successfully. In refractory cases, injection and replacement of the herniated fat may be worth a trial.

9

The Hip Region

Localized tender points and trigger points are found frequently in the abundant musculature and fibrous tissues over and about the hip joint. Similar diagnostic and therapeutic considerations prevail for these disorders as at the low back and elsewhere. The inflamed or irritated articular synovium and/or periarticular, secondary sites of irritation (and inflammation?), may produce the pain and tenderness adjacent to the joint. Rheumatoid, degenerative, posttraumatic or other arthropathy may be responsible. Soft tissue lesions and bursitis occur over and near the hip as in other locations.

PERIARTICULAR INJECTIONS

Localized superficial and deep tenderness about the hip is likely to be associated with some limitation of motion. Injection of the sore points may prove helpful, posteriorly about the greater trochanter, at one or more circumscribed points of tenderness. The injections are given deeply with a 2 or 2½ in., 22-G needle, 10 ml of 0.5 to 1 per cent lidocaine at each tender point. When effective, increasing intervals of comfort should follow. Otherwise, prednisolone suspension, 10 to 20 mg, is added.

BURSAL INJECTIONS

Inflammation and calcification of bursae about the hips joint may cause symptoms. When a bursa is calcified, it is readily located by X-ray films. If it is accessible, as in trochanteric bursitis, needling, aspiration, and injection with analgesic-corticosteroid preparation may be beneficial. At

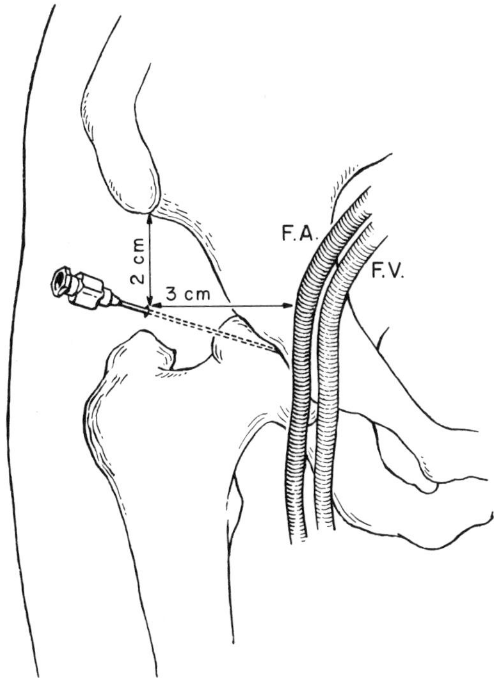

Fig. 9–1. Anterior approach for arthrocentesis of the hip joint.

times, the presumed bursitis or visualized bursal calcification is deep and not readily reached by needling, but when accessible, treatment by injection may be effective.

Trochanteric bursitis may occur especially over the greater trochanter with acute, subacute, or chronic symptoms. Pain arises from resting on the side of the hip; tenderness to palpation is localized sharply over the greater trochanter. Abduction of the hip and internal rotation are uncomfortable.

This localization is demonstrable and accessible to injection with corticosteroid, 25 to 50 mg of prednisolone suspension with 3 to 10 ml of lidocaine.

ARTHROCENTESIS OF THE HIP

The hip joint is the largest in the body, but it is usually the most difficult to enter and to aspirate. It has a dense capsule, enclosed by large ligaments and abundant, soft connective tissues. Pathologic joints may have overriding hypertrophic changes and inflamed joints may have greatly thickened synovia. If the joint architecture is greatly disturbed,

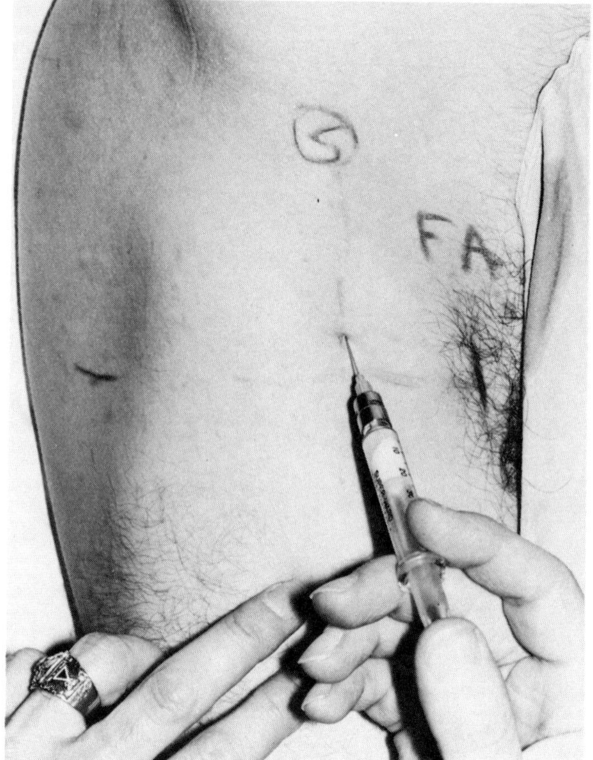

Fig. 9–2. Anterior arthrocentesis and injection of the hip joint.

it may be impossible to enter the joint space. Aspiration of fluid signaling actual entry of the synovial cavity with a needle is uncommon. Injection is carried out whether fluid is obtained or not. Accordingly results are unpredictable.

The joint may be entered and injected by the anterior or lateral approach. By the anterior method the patient lies supine with the extremity straight and slightly rotated externally. After suitable cleansing and a skin wheal, a 20-G needle, 2.5 to 4 in. long (according to the patient's size) is used. The entry is made at a point 2 cm below the anterior superior spine of the ilium and 3 cm lateral to the palpated femoral pulse, approximately at the level of the upper edge of the greater trochanter (Figs. 9–1 and 9–2). The needle is directed at an angle of 60°, posteriorly and medially, penetrating the tough capsular ligaments to bone. The needle then is withdrawn slightly and aspiration is attempted (Hollander, 1966; Miller, 1957; Findler & Post). Occasionally, fluid is obtained. In any case the joint is then injected with 25 to 50 mg of prednisolone suspension, to which 2 to 3 ml of 1 per cent lidocaine may be added.

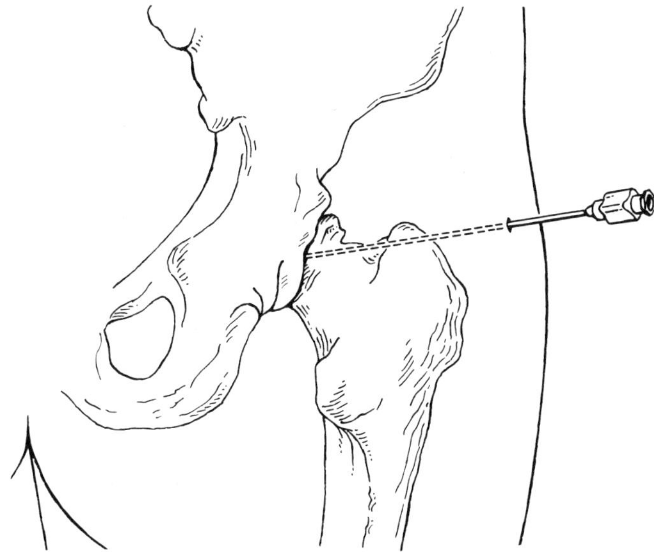

Fig. 9–3. Lateral approach for arthrocentesis of the hip joint.

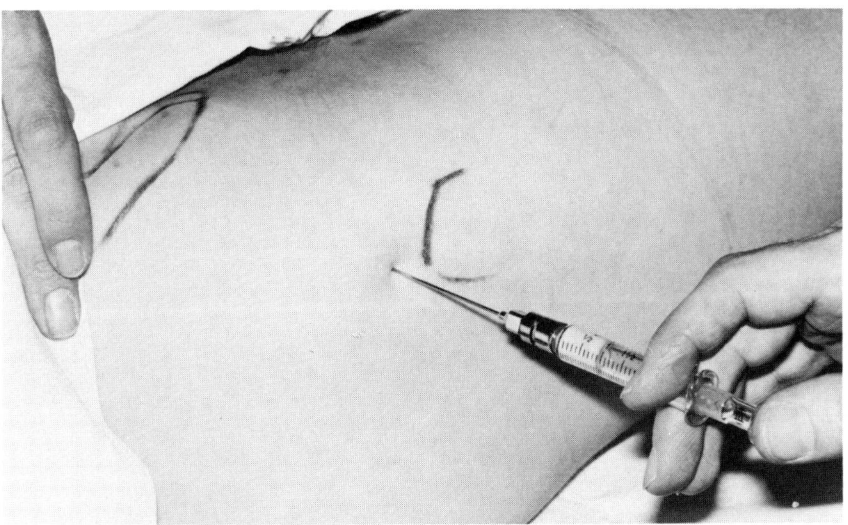

Fig. 9–4. Lateral arthrocentesis and injection of the hip joint.

Injection of the hip joint by the lateral route is simpler only in that the needle follows the line of the femoral neck to the articulation (Hollander, 1966; Miller, 1957) (Figs. 9–3 and 9–4). It is difficult to be sure of the entry through the capsule into the joint space here too, because only occasionally is fluid aspirated.

The greater trochanter of the femur is palpated (having the patient rotate the limb, if necessary). With the limb outwardly rotated, a wheal is made just anterior to the greater trochanter. A 22- or 20-G, 3- to 4.0-in. needle is directed medially (walked) along the neck of the femur, toward a point below the middle of the inguinal ligament to a depth of 2.5 to 3.5 in., until the joint capsule is reached and penetrated. Aspiration is carried out, if possible, and the medication is injected through the intact needle, after changing syringes. The dosage is the same as by the anterior approach.

The femoral (as well as the humeral) head has been an occasional site of osteonecrosis due to repeated, frequent introduction of corticosteroids. Intraarticular injection at this location, as elsewhere, should be repeated at no closer intervals than 4 weeks, preferably 6 to 12 weeks with due consideration for the possibility of so-called steroid arthropathy.

10

The Lower Limb

THE THIGH

Occasionally painful soft tissue lesions occur in the thigh. Trauma, strain, and muscular localization of systemic or local disorders often are responsible. Treatment then follows the usual management of such disturbances of soft tissues. Poor posture, arthropathy, neurologic disorders, old fractures, or local strain may be responsible. The basic disturbance should receive customary corrective attention.

Injections. The methods used in soft tissue lesions are applied here in localization and injection.

THE KNEE AREA

The chief structures requiring injection in the knee area are: tender points; ligamentary, tendinous, and other forms of periarthritis; bursitis; synovitis with or without definitive arthritis; meniscal cysts, and popliteal (Baker's) cysts.

PERIARTHRITIS

When tender points are found (with no cutaneous hyperesthesia), or soreness is provoked by certain motions, local traumatic or inflammatory disorder is suggested. These complaints may arise from strained or injured periarticular tissues, tendons, and ligaments, especially at their insertions and attachments.

Tender points to deep palpation about the knee occur at the medial or lateral condyle or at either side of the tibial head, occasionally at the head of the fibula. These may be injected with 3 to 5 ml of 1% Xylocaine, at one or more sore points. Repeated, longer intervals of response warrant a series of injections. If the relief is brief but definite, 10 to 15 mg of prednisolone suspension should then be injected with the analgesic solution.

Medial tendinitis or lateral tendinitis of the knee may be encountered, with tenderness and uncomfortable mobility. Sometimes a bursa with or without calcification forms at the medial or lateral collateral ligament of the knee, producing pain and point tenderness, increased by specific movements of the joint to one side or the other. Local infiltration is frequently effective with small amounts of lidocaine (1 to 3 ml) and/or the addition of prednisolone suspension (10 to 25 mg).

Tenderness at the collateral ligament at either side of the knee may be striking, as at the medial side in the Pellegrini-Stieda syndrome.

BURSITIS

Prepatellar bursitis, swelling and effusion of the bursa overlying the patella, is an obvious abnormality. The bursal reaction often is traumatic or the result of repetitive provocative activity. Tenderness will depend on the degree of inflammation. The possibility of infection must be considered. Aspiration yields clear, serous fluid usually; then with or without 1 ml of lidocaine 10 to 25 mg of prednisolone suspension are instilled. In some cases the procedure may need to be repeated once or a few times for a lasting effect, provided any provocative activity is eliminated.

Suprapatellar bursitis is associated usually with synovitis. Occasionally, when the bursa is largely separated developmentally or otherwise from the synovial cavity with a slight communication, effusion is especially prominent at the suprapatellar area.

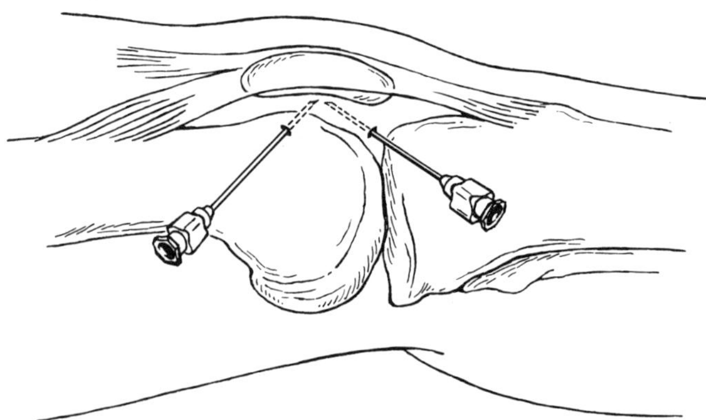

Fig. 10–1. Medial arthrocentesis of the knee joint, showing the usual entry site.

Other bursae are less common in this location, but adventitious developments occur. Fluctuation or point prominence and tenderness due to effusion present the best site of entry for aspiration and injection.

ARTHROCENTESIS OF THE KNEE JOINT

The knee, with the largest synovial space in the body, is the most frequently aspirated joint. Its painful involvement produces visible or palpable effusions making it easy to enter and to inject. When a large effusion occurs, any fluctuant point or bulge is likely to be an adequate entry site. When a small amount of fluid is present, the entry into the synovial space is somewhat more difficult. In any case the most efficient procedure is apt to be a standard technique.

Aspiration of the knee joint is done with the patient lying supine on a table with the lower extremities as fully extended as possible. The site of entry is just below the point where a horizontal line tangential to the upper margin of the patella crosses another paralleling the medial or lateral border cephalad (Figs. 10–1 and 10–2). From 25 to 62.5 mg of prednisolone suspension, or equivalent, may be administered through the intact needle after aspiration.

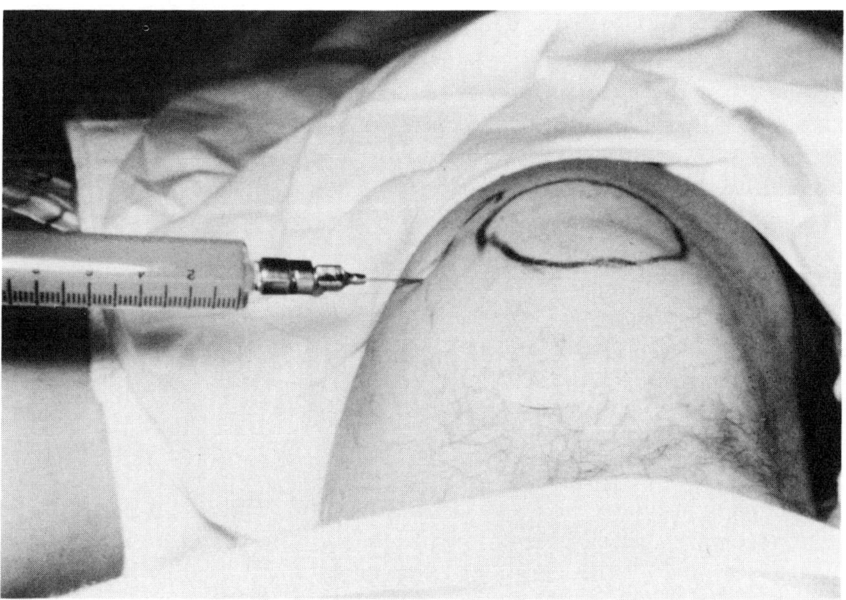

Fig. 10–2. Arthrocentesis of the knee joint.

The most commonly used entrance is at the anteromedial side where a larger space is palpable between the patella and the medial condyle. At the point of entry, after cleansing and aseptic preparation of the skin, a wheal is made. The needle (2-in., 20-G) may be directed downward or upward and laterally to advance into the joint space under the patella. When cartilage is touched, once the needle is in the synovial space, it signifies that the needle has proceeded far enough, especially if fluid is aspirated.

The lateral approach to the knee is sometimes used. It is especially convenient for a suprapatellar effusion. The point of penetration is at the point where a line tangential to the upper border of the patella crosses another paralleling the lateral border. The needle is directed medially and downward (or upward) to advance into the joint space under the patella, or into the greatest bulge of the effusion.

The infrapatellar route is used chiefly in the presence of a contracture of the joint or ankylosis of the patella. With the knee flexed, the needle is inserted through a skin wheal at either side of the inferior patellar tendon through or above the infrapatellar fat pad. It is directed under the patella into the joint, advancing between the femoral condyles. Fluid is difficult to obtain with this approach. After aspiration, 1 ml of lidocaine with 25 mg of prednisolone suspension is instilled into the joint space.

Popliteal (Baker's) cyst may occur in the popliteal space as an adventitious structure arising from tendon sheath or extraarticular connective tissue. In an adult a significant popliteal cyst is almost invariably rheumatoid in origin. The prominence often is a posterior capsular herniation of the synovium. With aspiration the cyst collapses, when it does not communicate with the capsule of the knee. After aspiration, 20 to 25 mg of prednisolone suspension with or without a local anesthetic is introduced. If the cyst is secondary to synovitis of the knee with posterior herniation or rupture of the synovium, the cyst usually recurs. Synovectomy should be considered in these cases.

If aspiration and injection must be repeated, an interval of 4 to 12 weeks should elapse. Undue repetition may damage the joint (Bently; Sweetman).

DISORDERS OF LEG MUSCLES

Trauma or strain of the leg muscles is not rare. When acute, it is likely to be recognized readily. Acute or subacute pain in the posterior muscles of the leg may cause disabling discomfort unrelieved by the usual measures. Weak feet may or may not be associated. Deep venous lesions must be excluded.

Strain of the achilles tendon and its muscular attachments may be the

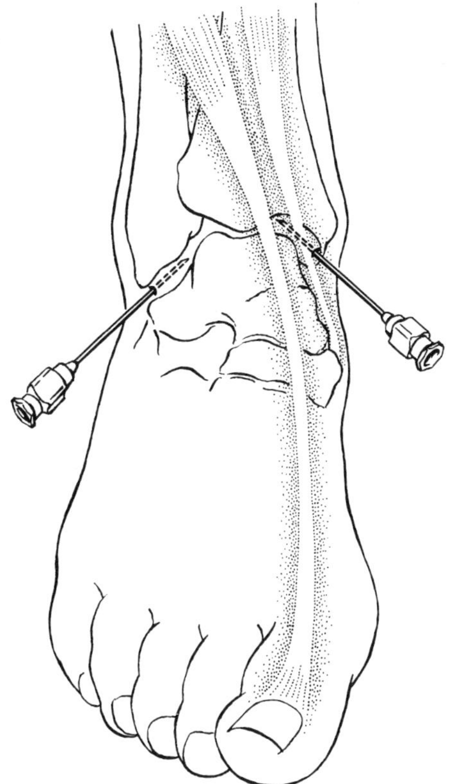

Fig. 10–3. Arthrocentesis of the ankle joint (medial or lateral compartment).

cause of acute pain in the calf. The ecchymosis of trauma may not be presented. No signs of venous or arterial involvement are demonstrable. Sharply localized deep tenderness is obtained. Orthopedic measures prove helpful.

Achilles bursitis, as well as other bursal involvement, may appear at the ankle and foot. Aspiration and/or lidocaine injection, and later lidocaine and prednisolone may be introduced. These procedures should be carefully considered, insofar as spontaneous rupture of the achilles tendon has occurred in patients with rheumatoid arthritis, ankylosing spondylitis, and systemic lupus who have received steroid injections into the achilles bursal area (Sweetman; Rajakumer).

PERSISTENT POINT TENDERNESS AT THE LOWER EXTREMITY

Other sites of persistent soreness circumscribed at any of the muscles of the thigh or leg may represent previous trauma or localized inflamma-

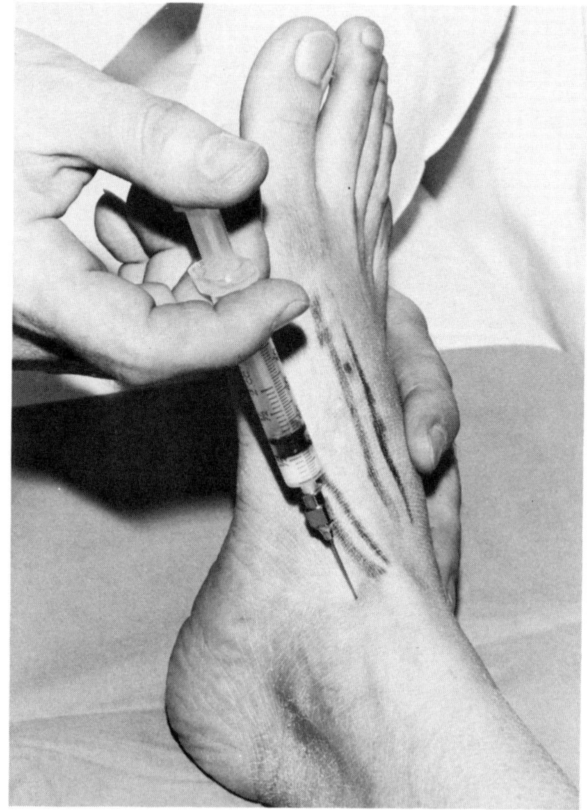

Fig. 10–4. Arthrocentesis and injection of the ankle joint.

tion. If unresponsive to standard measures, palpable tender points are readily injected (avoiding veins and arteries). After aspiration, the injection is given at the point of tenderness, with a 22-G needle (1.5 to 2.0 in.) with lidocaine 2 to 5 ml (1%) alone as a test, then with 10 to 25 mg of prednisolone suspension added. The procedure may have to be repeated within 1 to 4 weeks.

ARTHROCENTESIS OF THE ANKLE JOINT

The ankle joint is frequently difficult to enter. The foot is held in slight plantar flexion (Brewerton). After identifying the extensor hallucis longus tendon, the usual point of entry is just medial to it, approximately 1 cm above and 1 cm lateral to the internal (medial) malleolus. The needle is directed toward the tibioastragalar (talar) articulation, somewhat laterally from the internal malleolus (Figs. 10–3 and 10–4). Lidocaine may be used first, injecting as the needle advances until it reaches the joint space. Then aspiration is carried out. The syringe is changed to introduce 20 to 30 mg of prednisolone suspension with or without additional lidocaine (1%).

Sometimes tenderness and swelling are largely noted about and below the lateral malleolus at the ankle. Entry then is directed at the lateral portion of the joint in a similar manner.

ARTHROCENTESIS OF TARSAL AND TARSOMETATARSAL JOINTS

Occasionally, localized pain, swelling, and tenderness to palpation require injection of the tarsal and metatarsal joints. Circumscribed tenderness, sometimes overlying swelling, localize the point of entry.

A 24-G needle is used to enter the dorsal surface. It is teased between the tarsal bones into the desired space until it moves freely. Fluid sometimes is aspirated. A dose of 10 to 15 mg of prednisolone with or without 0.25 ml of lidocaine should flow without resistance. Injection subcutaneously at the tender point may suffice.

INJECTION OF METATARSOPHALANGEAL JOINTS

Swelling and point tenderness at any metatarsophalangeal joint is best determined by palpation at the dorsum of the foot or in the plantar space under the toes at the distal surface of the metatarsal arch. The affected joints can thereby be readily identified. This distal plantar metatarsal surface at its upper portion provides a sheltered point of injection for the affected articulations (Fig. 10–5*A*). The approach often is made at the dorsal surface (Fig. 10–5*B*).

Through a wheal, the solution of 0.5 ml of lidocaine (1%) with 10 to 20 mg prednisolone is deposited into or over the affected joint. An ethyl chloride spray may be used in place of the wheal.

Tenderness of these joints may be felt also at the dorsal (extensor) surface of the foot. The joints may be injected by that route. Traction on the toe to be injected may facilitate insertion of the needle.

The first metatarsophalangeal joint may be the site of acute or chronic synovitis. It may be entered through a medial dorsal approach by teasing with a 24-G needle; 10 to 20 mg of prednisolone suspension may be injected (Fig. 10–6*A*). Subcutaneous entry of the swollen capsule for aspiration and injection, or deposit of the dosage over the joint space is usually sufficient.

Bursitis overlying this joint at its medial surface is common. Due to

A

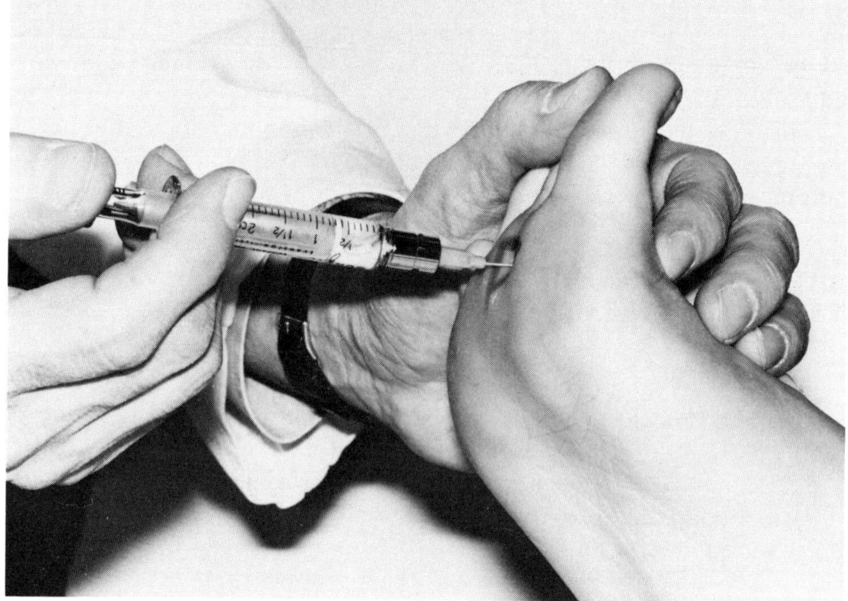

B

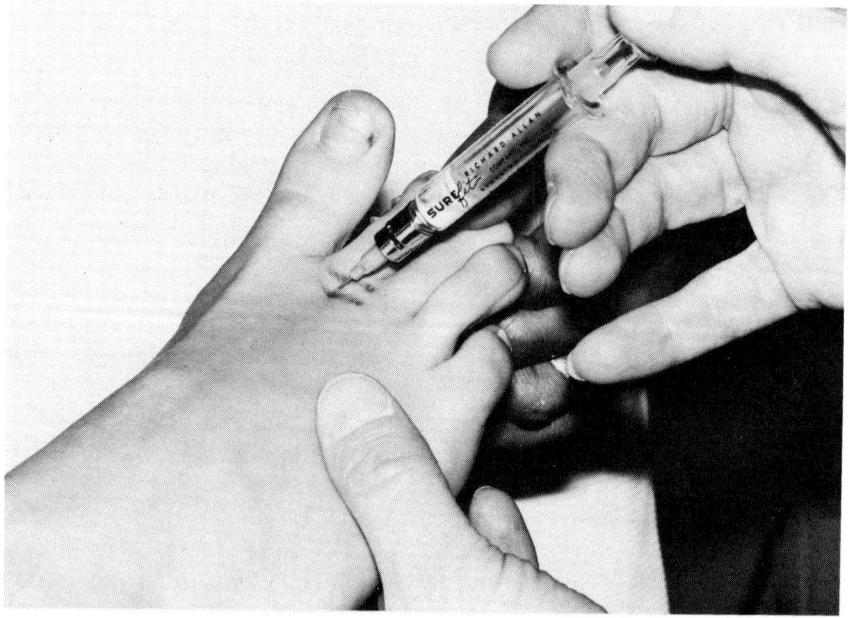

Fig. 10–5. *A.* Arthrocentesis and injection or periarticular infiltration of the metatarsophalangeal joint at the distal plantar prominence. *B.* The dorsal approach to the metatarsophalangeal joint.

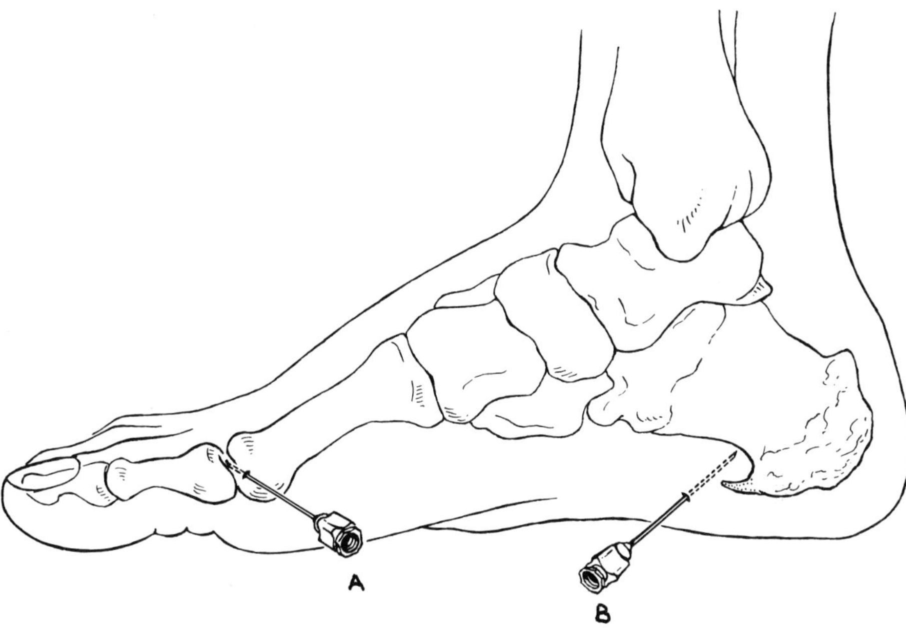

Fig. 10–6. *A*. Arthrocentesis and injection of the first metatarsophalangeal joint. *B*. Injection of the painful heel (plantar fasciitis or bursitis).

trauma, infection may develop. Aspiration of the bursal effusion gives relief (the aspirate should be cultured). Orthopedic corrections or special shoes may maintain it. If no infection is present, and if swelling recurs rapidly, the bursa is injected with 5 to 10 mg of prednisolone suspension.

CALCANEAL BURSITIS

In calcaneal bursitis, mechanical factors should be looked for. A calcaneal spur may be associated. Orthopedic shoe corrections and aids are often sufficient treatment.

A sharply demarcated tender spot is located at the midpoint of the anterior or inferior calcaneal border in the plantar area. This point is marked and continued in a transverse line to the medial plantar surface of the foot (Fig. 10–6*B*). At this point a 1 to 2-in., 22- or 24-G needle is directed laterally and slightly upward and dorsally to slide into the space at the midpoint of the calcaneus. The introduction of 1 ml of lidocaine with 10 to 25 mg of prednisolone suspension is then carried out.

The Dermo-Jet or Hypospray permits a more gentle injection at the tarsal, metatarsal, and other joints of the toes.

11

Management of Musculoskeletal Disorders

Most painful, localized disturbances of the locomotor system are of mild traumatic, irritative, possibly transient inflammatory origin. Often they are self-limiting or responsive to simple medical and/or physical measures (See Table 9, page 95).

We are concerned here with conditions that are acute and require rapid relief, or with the less severe but troublesome discomfort and disability that persist in spite of the patient's self-care or the physician's recommendations. Some acute disorders demand immediate medical intervention; these include acute calcareous tendinitis of the shoulder or bursitis, acute sciatica or radiculitis, acute synovitis, and similar disturbances.

In many of these conditions—with the patient's cooperation—simple, basic measures may permit a more tolerable level of symptoms, although full recovery may take longer.

The use of systemic medications and other methods of management often help to minimize the course of symptoms or reduce the number of injections required.

Certainly in less compelling circumstances, basic methods of management, including the choice of the analgesic adequate to control the pain. should be given a sufficient trial. The various items constituting the basic program should be discussed (see Table 9, page 95). Many uncomfortable musculoskeletal disorders respond to a suitable combination of measures. (Neustadt 1971)

Rest of a painful part, with a support or splint if necessary is a fundamental aid in management. For multiple, painful sites, especially at the

TABLE 9. Basic Measures in Painful Articular and Musculoskeletal Disorders

Rest of painful part, or whole body
Analgesics
- salicylates
- acetaminophen
- propoxyphene (Darvon), or ethoheptazine compounds (Zactane)
- phenylbutazone (Butazolidin)
- oxyphenbutazone (Tandearil)
- indomethacin (Indocin)
- codeine or meperidine (Demerol) for acute, severe symptoms
- pentozacine (Talwin) for continuing discomfort

Corticosteroids (rarely, brief courses)
Relaxants or barbiturates for synergistic or specific effects
Physical therapy (heat, cold, electrical modalities, exercises)
Mechanical aids (splints, supports, bed board)
Psychotherapy
Treatment of underlying or associated conditions

lower extremities, and certainly if a systemic condition is the source, a period of complete bed rest may be indicated.

When poor body mechanics, atypical features, or special structural problems are associated with unresponsive pain and disability, an orthopedic consultation may be helpful.

In patients who are obviously emotionally disturbed, or in those who present bizarre symptoms unrelieved or worsened by basic measures, a neuropsychiatric evaluation should be considered.

In the paragraphs below we will consider the various forms of basic management usually preceding, sometimes accompanying, the local injection of painful, circumscribed locomotor disorders.

SYSTEMIC THERAPY VS. LOCAL INJECTION

It is usually preferable to control complaints by oral, systemic medications, when possible, rather than by local analgesic injections. However, acute disabling symptoms, demanding quick relief, such as calcific tendinitis, acute synovitis with effusion and other conditions mentioned above are exceptions. Therefore, the search for improved oral pharmacologic agents—analgesics, antiinflammatory compounds, muscular relaxants, etc.—continues.

SYSTEMIC MEDICATIONS

In the authors' opinion more versatile and effective control of painful disorders has been provided by the advent of the corticosteroids, butazones (phenylbutazone and oxyphenbutazone), propoxyphene (Darvon) and ethoheptazine (Zactane), indomethacin (Indocin), and in selected cases, the so-called muscle relaxants.

Any of these preparations, or combinations of them, may prove helpful. Nevertheless, there are conditions in which localized joint inflammation or circumscribed musculoskeletal pain and disability prove resistant to systemic pharmacologic therapy and physical modalities. These disorders are suitable for local or regional injection. Apart from salicylates, narcotics, and corticoids, any ill effects of the newer preparations during pregnancy are not well documented. The dosage for children must be worked out individually. The pharmaceutical compounds will be considered in the following paragraphs. Standard medications and physical methods are advocated whenever possible.

Salicylates

We regard acetylsalicylic acid as the simplest, most effective analgesic when given in adequate doses—5 to 25 grains (0.3 to 1.5 g) every 4 hours when awake. It may be used alone or in combination with other analgesics. For patients with chronic or recurrent pain problems, we prescribe buffered acetylsalicylic acid during or after meals and at bedtime. In some patients who object to "the same medicine," it may be necessary to prescribe another form of the many different salicylate preparations. Acetylsalicylic acid in sustained release formulation, taken at bedtime, may in some cases provide a longer duration of nocturnal relief. Patients are advised to drink a full glass of liquid with each salicylate dose to avoid gastrointestinal symptoms.

When gastric intolerance of mild degree is provoked by acetylsalicylic acid, the "coated" preparations such as Ecotrin and Enseals or enteric-coated sodium salicylate or salicylamide tablets may be substituted. In the presence of gastritis, or of a gastric or duodenal ulcer, the latter compound, the amide of salicylic acid (not a true salicylate), may be the only drug related to salicylates likely to be tolerated. Calcium or aluminum salicylate are occasionally tolerated and effective when acetylsalicylic acid and sodium salicylate are not.

In addition to gastric irritation, the symptoms of salicylism or alkalosis may be produced by large dosage. These reactions subside when the dosage is reduced. Gastric bleeding sometimes occurs, and must be watched for. Decreased hearing ability requires a reduction of dosage or a change to another analgesic.

Propoxyphene and Ethoheptazine

Propoxyphene (Darvon) is probably a useful analgesic prescribed in doses of 32 to 65 mg. Ethoheptazine (Zactane), an analogous formulation, may be used in doses of 75 mg. In adequate doses, they appear to be effective analgesics for musculoskeletal pain. Although approximating codeine in composition, action, and usefulness, they are not classed as narcotics in this country. In any dosage these compounds are best taken during meals with food and at bedtime with milk or antacid. For severe, unresponsive pain we may rarely give up to eight capsules of Darvon-65 in 24 hours, until improvement; and then gradually reduce the dosage. This also applies to Zactane which approximates Darvon in effectiveness. A new formulation of propoxyphene (Darvon-N), recently made available, allows stable liquid dosage forms. The pharmacologic properties are similar to those of Darvon; however owing to molecular weight differences, a dose of 100 mg of Darvon-N is required for an effective equivalent to that of 65 mg of Darvon.

Reactions. Darvon or Zactane may produce drowsiness, dizziness, or lightheadedness in some subjects. Nausea, indigestion, or gastric disturbance may occur unless the drug is taken with food, milk, or antacid, when these reactions are occasional. If such side-effects persist, the preparation is stopped. Constipation is a not infrequent complaint. Sometimes cutaneous eruptions and other evidence of sensitivity may occur. The medication then should be discontinued. Drug dependence, possible habituation or addiction has been reported in sporadic cases.

Phenylbutazone

Phenylbutazone (Butazolidin, Butazolidin-Alka) is an established analgesic for a variety of musculoskeletal pains. It has some antiinflammatory action. When simpler drugs do not suffice, it is often an effective agent in doses of 100 mg during meals and at bedtime with milk. The Butazolidin-Alka capsule, like the tablet of plain Butazolidin, comes in a 100-mg capsule, but contains aluminum hydroxide gel. It may be administered in doses of 300 to 600 mg daily for 7 to 10 days. If no relief occurs, it is stopped.

When the pain is abolished, the dose is decreased gradually daily until the drug is discontinued. In chronic, painful conditions responsive to phenylbutazone, such as ankylosing spondylitis, we have prescribed it in regular maintenance dosage for a number of years, with regular periodic clinical and laboratory observations (blood and urine). Absence of reactions in the early phase of administration, as with other drugs, is no guarantee that untoward effects may not develop later.

Oxyphenbutazone (Tandearil), an analog of phenylbutazone, is probably as effective as phenylbutazone, and may give a somewhat lesser frequency of reactions. Some clinicians prefer it. The indications and contraindications are similar to those for phenylbutazone.

Reactions. The most frequent side-effects are cutaneous eruptions, gastric irritation, ulcerogenic symptoms, and peripheral edema. Hemodilution with lowered hemoglobin and erythrocyte count may occur temporarily and disappear with continued therapy. Old duodenal ulcers may be reactivated. In severe hypertension, cardiac insufficiency, hepatic or renal disease, and in those with a history of gastric or duodenal ulcer the drug is contraindicated. Agranulocytosis, generalized allergic reactions, stomatitis, salivary gland enlargement may occur.

These compounds may enhance the effect of anticoagulants although ordinarily they do not of themselves accelerate antiprothrombin activity. They also may potentiate sulfonylureas, other sulfonamide preparations, and insulin. If for any reason concomitant therapy with such drugs is carried out, due precautions must be taken.

When we prescribe butazone compounds, we perform a complete blood count and urinalysis weekly or every 2 weeks for dosage of 300 mg or more a day, and every 3 to 8 weeks for lesser dosage taken regularly. During many years of observing butazone treatment the authors have not seen any fatal or serious incidents, excepting occasional episodes of gastrointestinal bleeding.

Indomethacin

Indomethacin (Indocin) reportedly is effective in some inflammatory, degenerative, and other painful musculoskeletal disorders. When simplier drugs fail to relieve pain, this preparation is worthy of a trial.

The authors prescribe one capsule (25 mg) the first day with breakfast, adding one capsule daily or every few days with each meal, and a fourth capsule at bedtime with milk or a snack. Administered in this manner, early untoward reactions are greatly reduced. If necessary, the dosage may be increased gradually to 50 mg during or after meals. When a level of comfort has been maintained for an adequate time, the dosage is reduced gradually to a daily maintenance amount of 25 to 100 mg.

Reactions. The side-effects most commonly seen with this compound are headache, lightheadedness, dizziness, and gastrointestinal disturbances such as anorexia, nausea, vomiting, abdominal discomfort and diarrhea. If side-effects occur, the medication should be reduced or stopped, and then resumed in the lowest dosage which was previously tolerated, after the unwanted effects have disappeared. If the undesirable reactions recur, the drug is withdrawn.

Indocin may activate an old peptic ulcer or possibly provoke new ulcer disease. It is contraindicated in patients with a history of gastric or duodenal ulcer, gastritis, and ulcerative colitis. Gastrointestinal bleeding without demonstrable ulceration may occur. Abnormalities in liver function tests and a rise in blood urea nitrogen may develop rarely. The frequency of side-effects is greater in the aging, calling for special caution in prescribing Indocin for elderly patients.

Indocin must be used cautiously in patients with a history, or symptoms, of a neuropsychiatric disorder, parkinsonism, or epilepsy.

Other Medications

Acetaminophen (Tylenol, Nebs, Tempra) is a mild analgesic suitable chiefly for patients who react adversely to the salicylates or other analgesics, or for those with complications, such as peptic ulcer or gastric irritability. It does not influence prothrombin time. The dosage for adults is one or two 300 mg tablets, 3 or 4 times a day, after meals and at bedtime.

Acetaminophen has rarely been proved to produce any side-effects or adverse reactions, such as gastric discomfort. Renal irritation, evidenced by proteinuria, occurs rarely.

Narcotics are justified for temporary use to relieve severe pain, especially in acute bursitis, radiculitis, trauma, and even in attacks of gout or arthritis. The strongest dose usually required is a hypodermic injection of 75 mg of meperidine (Demerol), every 4 to 8 hours for one or two doses. Ordinarily, codeine sulfate per os, 15 to 30 mg, usually given with acetylsalicylic acid 4 times a day until relieved, will suffice.

Pentozacine (Talwin) is the latest "nonnarcotic" analgesic. We have used it effectively in patients with refractory musculoskeletal or arthritic symptoms, but it is not always well tolerated. In view of its brief clinical trial, it must be used cautiously. A few reports already have appeared to indicate habituation (Wolfe *et al.*).

Talwin is available in 1-ml vials (30 mg) for parenteral use and as a 50-mg tablet for oral administration.

In our limited experience with Talwin, we have encountered dizziness, lightheadedness, and/or nausea. We are impressed by the tolerance shown by some previously reactive patients, when the dose is worked up gradually from 0.25 to 1.0 ml intramuscularly 1 to 3 times a day (every 8 hours) or one-half tablet a day perorally, increased slowly to one tablet 2 to 4 times a day. There remains an impressive percentage of patients who do not get relief, even when they have acquired tolerance. These observations on tolerance and adverse reactions apply with varying emphasis to nearly all of the analgesics discussed here. Even if mild lightheadedness occurs, Talwin has been found useful for controlling nocturnal pain in some patients.

Corticosteroids

Corticosteroids and corticotropin are potent analgesics chiefly by virtue of their antiinflammatory effects, their mobilization of inflammatory edema fluid, resolution of cellular infiltration, and other actions. Their regular administration perorally or intramuscularly for a limited time may be indicated to quickly terminate attacks of acute arthritis, bursitis (tenosynovitis), or gout. These compounds also may be employed as a final resort for the troublesome, multiple pains of systemic conditions, such as polyarthritis, and in suitable doses for some time in polymyositis, polymyalgia rheumatica, polyarteritis, or systemic lupus.

If a patient presents no contraindications, and other medications have failed, a systemic corticoid is worth a trial. Prednisone or its equivalent may be prescribed in doses of 10 to 20 mg a day. It should be reduced gradually and withdrawn in 2 to 3 weeks when used to eliminate localized myalgia, arthralgia, bursitis or synovitis.

Corticosteroid suspensions are injected locally at the site of circumscribed pain of suspected inflammatory origin in many specific conditions. They are given by local injection with analgesic solution of lidocaine or corticosteroid suspension (or as a mixture of both). This approach is logical, faster, and carries less potential for adverse reactions.

The relative contraindications and adverse reactions to corticosteroids are well known and do not require detailed discussion here. Common contraindications include diabetes mellitus, active or arrested tuberculosis or other systemic or local infection, psychosis, peptic ulcer disease or osteoporosis. Even when corticoids are given as depot injections, some systemic absorption occurs (10 to 30% depending on the compound). Regular observations for certain physical signs and laboratory tests are mandatory during continued local or systemic administration.

The spacing of corticosteroid injections, especially when given into joints, is important. Intraarticular injections in most cases should probably not be repeated more often than at intervals of 4 to 12 weeks, the longer the intervals the better. Local injections must be given at intervals unlikely to produce undesirable side-effects. Aseptic or osteonecrosis is a potential hazard of repeated local administration, as well as systemic, and is being reported more frequently. Iatrogenic infection is avoided by meticulous cleanliness and asepsis.

Numerous proprietary analgesic preparations and combinations can be found in *Physicians' Desk Reference* and *AMA Drug Evaluations.* Undoubtedly, many of these would prove to be useful in the control of pain. The authors do not prescribe combinations of analgesic compounts routinely in a single "shotgun" preparation, owing to the difficulty of assessing the role of each ingredient in providing relief, or in causing an adverse reaction. It is also difficult to adjust dosage for individual substances included in it.

Relaxants, Tranquilizers, Sedatives

Systemic and muscular relaxants, tranquilizers, and sedatives are useful in treating tense or anxious individuals. Generally, they are employed as supplements to salicylates and the other analgesics.

Meprobamate, in doses of 200 to 400 mg 2 to 4 times a day, may be prescribed for its mild peripheral (muscle-relaxing) effect, as well as any other tranquilizer with similar action. Some so-called relaxants—Norflex, Robaxin, Paraflex and, more recently, Maolate—have been proposed for this purpose. The authors have not been notably impressed by the specificity of the latter preparations given alone for presumed muscular spasm and its associated pain, but such benefits have been reported. Diazepam (Valium) has been found recently to be effective for mild muscle spasms and reducing tension.

A soporific at bedtime to supplement analgesics is desirable until adequate pain relief is achieved.

The Therapeutic Attitude

Learning to live and cope with some discomfort is a helpful therapeutic attitude to be cultivated by patients with chronic musculoskeletal disease. The physician should make it clear to his patients that the complete abolition of chronic pain by potent drugs is a hazardous undertaking. The larger dosages required increase the possibility of adverse side-effects from analgesic and antiinflammatory agents. The pharmacy and medication cannot entirely replace sound philosophy and motivation.

Other Considerations

Habituation may occur with narcotics, of course. The "addictive"-like qualities of corticosteroids are reflected in patients in whom it is difficult, or sometimes seemingly impossible, to cut down or stop the corticoid. Whether their difficulties are due to "physiologic habituation" is another question.

The possibility of habituation to synthetic formulations with narcotic-like structures such as Darvon, Zactane, and the more recently introduced Talwin is moot. They are listed as nonnarcotics on the basis of authoritative observations, but addictive experiences have been reported in a small number. Codeine, of course, may become habit-forming. Over many years we have seen it happen only once in a patient with the "habituation personality" and a history of a drug habit not previously admitted.

The dependence of the pain-driven patient on analgesics, relaxants, or sedatives must be borne in mind and excesses explained and prevented.

Justifiable habituation may be rarely indicated in patients with painful syndromes or arthritis refractory to available measuers when serious medical complications are associated, and also in the elderly, when surgical intervention is not feasible. In such situations it is justifiable and humane to risk the use of regular doses of codeine or other narcotics as a final therapeutic resort. Some understanding with the family and the patient is desirable.

Injections, or parenteral therapies, impose another responsibility. Many individuals become apprehensive when faced with an injection and their fears should be allayed. Before prescribing oral medication it is important to establish potential hypersensitivity; this holds especially for parenteral preparations. A careful therapeutic history should elicit information on past reactions to such preparations as procaine, narcotics, and even corticosteroid suspensions.

The needle-shy, apprehensive patient will cooperate better if he is recognized beforehand and dealt with gently. Pain may be minimized by the use of ethyl chloride to freeze the skin, or by use of the newer instruments, such as the Dermo-Jet or Hypospray.

OTHER FORMS OF TREATMENT

X-radiation is rarely indicated in acute bursitis (tendinitis), especially of the shoulder, if the patient cannot or will not depend on analgesics to tide her over the acute period; or if she is needle-shy, or gets recurrent attacks despite responsiveness to injections, or presents significant contraindications to corticosteroids and butazone compounds. Subacute or chronic bursitis is treated with radiation for similar reasons. However the less acute the disorder, as a rule, the less likelihood of a good or satisfactory response. In patients in the sixth decade of life and older, the potential risk of a subsequent blood dyscrasia is not as important a consideration as it would be in patients in the younger age group.

Bursitis at the hip, when it is not amenable to local injection or usual measures, may respond to radiation.

Orthopedic devices must be considered for pain arising from trauma, or from disturbed body mechanics provoking articular or periarticular tissues. An elastic bandage, a wrist splint, or a surgical orthopedic corset (in low back pain) may play an important role in the therapeutic program. The use of specially made splints or moulds for painful or inflamed parts has recently been emphasized (Neustadt, 1971). Medications or injections often are doomed to failure, in any condition simultaneously requiring a support, if such a device is not prescribed and obtained. Orthopedic consultation and evaluation are helpful with these problems.

Surgery is indicated for some disturbances, which are intractable or recur in spite of other measures. These include injections, particularly for neural entrapment, persistent bursitis (especially calcific) of the shoulder, and for some discogenic disorders. Inadequately responsive inflammatory lesions of articular synovia, tendon sheaths, and bursae should be evaluated in consultation for surgical intervention. This step is indicated if two to three intrasynovial injections at well-spaced intervals fail to provide sustained control of symptoms.

Neurologic consultation may be useful when segmental or systemic neurologic features are suggested. Electromyography and other methods of electrodiagnosis in some muscular disorders, carpal tunnel syndrome, and others, may provide specific information.

Neurosurgical evaluation may be indicated, especially in refractory discogenic, radicular, or neural syndromes.

Neuropsychiatric evaluation and psychotherapy must be considered in chronic, unresponsive painful disorders with bizarre and unyielding complaints, especially when associated with anxiety states or depression.

Treatment of underlying or associated conditions, such as specific arthritides, diabetes, etc., must be continued. Local injection of lidocaine is not likely to provoke a systemic disease. When inflamed tissue is penetrated, a temporary reaction of local discomfort occasionally follows as the analgesic effect wears off (after-pain). The local introduction of corticosteroids must be carried out with due regard for any coexisting disease, and the possibility of provoking or aggravating it, such as diabetes, peptic ulcer, and others.

Cytotoxic compounds are being used systemically and by introduction into the affected synovium of inflamed joints. (Henderson and Nathan; Gristina *et al.*).

Other compounds, proposed for use as intra-articular therapy in persistent joint effusions, when conservative methods have failed, include phenylbutazone, osmium acid, radioactive gold and other radioactive agents (Neustadt & Steinbrocker, 1956; Hurri *et al.*; Makin & Robin; Oka *et al.*). The term chemical synovectomy has been introduced to describe the effects of the injection resulting from these potent agents. So far, this form of therapy is limited to investigative and experimental studies.

References

Bently, G. Disorganization of the knee, following intraarticular hydrocortisone injections. *J Bone Joint Surg 51-B*: 498, 1969.

Betcher, AM. A new technic for suprascapular nerve block. *Bull Hosp Joint Dis 10*: 233, 1949.

Bonica, JJ. *The Management of Pain.* Philadelphia, Lea & Febiger, 1953, p. 234.

Bonica, JJ. *Clinical Applications of Diagnostic and Therapeutic Nerve Blocks.* Springfield, Ill., Thomas, 1959.

Bonica, JJ. Nerve blocks for managing pain in the elderly, *Postgrad Med 47*: 215, 1964.

Breneman, JC. Five years experience with procaine-steroid injections. A diagnostic therapeutic tool for patients with low back pain. *J Occup Med 11*: 475, 1969.

Brewerton, DA. Pain in the ankle. *Brit Med J 3*: 99, 1969.

Brown, JH. Pressure intracaudal injection. *Med Times 89*: 1069, 1961.

Cassidy, JT and Bole, GG. Cutaneous atrophy secondary to intra-articular corticosteroid administration. *Ann Internal Med 65*: 1008–1018, (Nov) 1966.

Cohen, AS. *Laboratory Diagnostic Procedures in the Rheumatic Diseases.* Boston, Little, Brown & Co. 1967.

Copeman, WSC and Ackerman, WL. Fibrositis of the back. *Quart J Med 13*: 37, 1944.

Crisp, EJ and Kendall, PH. Treatment of periarthritis of the shoulder with hydrocortisone. *Brit Med J 1*: 1501, 1955.

Editorial. Local anesthetics for physicians and dentists. *The Medical Letter Drugs Ther 13*: 5, 1971.

Epstein, E. Triamcinolone in herpes zoster. *Consultant 2*: 53, 1972 (courtesy Waller, John).

Findler, JC and Post, M. Local injection therapy for rheumatic diseases. *JAMA 172*: 2021, 1960.

Findley, T and Patzer, R. The treatment of herpes zoster by paravertebral procaine block. *JAMA 128*: 1217, 1945.

Françon, F. A new clinical entity: ischial bursitis. *Rev Rhum 33*: 253, 1966.

Gage, M. Scalenus anticus syndrome, *Surg 5*: 599, 1939.

Gristina, AG, Pace, NA, Kantor, TG, and Thompson, WAL. Intra-articular thio-tepa compared with Depo-Medrol and procaine in the treatment of arthritis. *J Bone Joint Surg 52-A*: 1603, 1970.

Hannington-Kiff, JG. Treatment of intractable pain by Bupuvacaine nerve block. *Lancet 2*: 1392, 1971.

Henderson, ED and Nathan, FF. Experience with injection of nitrogen mustard into joints of patients with rheumatoid arthritis. *Southern Med J 62*: 1455, 1969.

Hollander, JL. Intrasynovial corticosteroid therapy. *In* Hollander, JL. *Arthritis*. Philadelphia, Lea & Febiger, 1966, p. 331.

Hollander, JL. Intrasynovial corticosteroid therapy in arthritis. *Maryland Med J 19*: 62, 1970.

Hurri, L, Sievers, K, and Oka, M. Intra-articular osmic acid in rheumatoid arthritis. *Acta Rheum Scand 9*: 20, 1963.

Labat, G. *Regional Anesthesia*, 2nd ed. Philadelphia, Saunders, 1928, p. 310.

McCarty, DJ and Hogan, JM. Inflammatory reaction after intra-synovial injection of microcrystaline adrenocorticosteroid esters. *Arth Rheum 7*: 359, 1964.

Makin, M and Robin, GC. Chronic synovial effusion treated with intra-articular radioactive gold. *JAMA 188*: 725, 1964.

Michele, AA, Davis, JJ, Krueger, FJ and Lichtor, JM. Scapulocostal syndrome. *NY J Med 50*: 1353, 1950.

Miller, JA. Joint paracentesis from an anatomic point of view. I. Shoulder, elbow, wrist and hand. *Surgery 40*: 993, 1956.

Miller, JA. Joint paracentesis from an anatomic point of view. II. Hip, knee, ankle and feet. *Surgery 41*: 999, 1957.

Murnaghan, GF and McIntosh, D. Hydrocortisone in painful shoulder. A controlled trial. *Lancet 2*: 798, 1955.

Neustadt, DH. *Chemistry and Therapy of Collagen Diseases*. Springfield, Ill., Thomas, 1963, p. 50.

Neustadt, DH. *Unpublished Data*

Neustadt, DH. Medical management of rheumatoid arthritis. *J. Albert Einstein Med Center 19*: 25, 1971.

Neustadt, DH and Steinbrocker, O. Observations on the effects of intra-articular phenylbutazone. *J. Lab Clin Med 47*: 284, 1956.

Oka, M, Rekonen, A, Ruotsi, A and Seppala, O. Intra-articular injection of Y-90 resin colloid in the treatment of rheumatoid knee joint effusions. *Acta Rheum Scand 17*: 148, 1971.

Phelan, GS. Soft tissue affections of the hand and wrist. *Hosp Med 7*: 47, 1971; The carpal tunnel syndrome. *J Bone Joint Surg 48-A*: 211, 1966.

Rajakumer, HK. Rupture of the patellar ligament after steroid infiltration. *J Bone Joint Surg 51-B*: 397, 1969.

Rome, ML. Treatment of bursitis, fibrositis and related conditions, in symposium and panel on recent therapeutic modalities. *NY J Med 62*: 2682, 1962.

Ropes, MW and Bauer, W. *Synovial Fluid Changes in Joint Disease.* Cambridge, Mass., Harvard Univ. Press (for Commonwealth Fund), 1953, p. 19.

Smith, DW. Stellate ganglion block. The tissue displacement method. *Amer J Surg 82*: 344, 1951.

Steinbrocker, O. *Arthritis in Modern Practice.* Philadelphia, Saunders, 1941, p. 345.

Steinbrocker, O. Local and regional analgesic injections in painful musculoskeletal disorders. *Arizona Med 9*: 27, 1952.

Steinbrocker, O, Neustadt, DH and Bosch, SJ. Painful shoulder syndromes. *Med Clin N Amer 39*: 1, 1955.

Steinbrocker, O. Management of some nonarticular rheumatic disorders. *Modern Treatm 1*: 1264, 1964.

Steinbrocker, O. An instrument for cutaneous wheals in hypersensitive and needle-shy subjects (the Dermo-Jet). *In preparation.*

Steinbrocker, O. Local corticosteroid injection therapy for idiopathic capsulitis of the shoulder (frozen shoulder). *In preparation.*

Sweetman, R. Corticosteroid arthropathy and tendon rupture. *J Bone Joint Surg 51-B*: 503, 1969.

Thompson, M. The elbow. *Brit Med J 3*: 399, 1969.

Travell, J and Bigelow, W. Role of somatic trigger areas in the patterns of hysteria. *Psychosom Med 9*: 333, 1945.

Wertheim, HM and Rovenstine, EA. Suprascapular nerve block. *Anesthesiology 2*: 541, 1941.

Wolfe, RC, Reidenberg, M, and Vispo, RH. Propoxyphene (Darvon) addiction and withdrawal syndrome. *Ann Int Med* 70, 1967.

Ziff, M, Contreres, V, and Schmid, TR. Use of the Hypospray jet injector for the intra-articular and local administration of hydrocortisone acetate. *Ann Rheum Dis 15*: 227, 1956.

Index

Page numbers in bold face indicate illustrations. Page numbers followed by the letter "t" indicate tabular information.

72 73 74 7 6 5 4 3 2 1